The Ethics
of
Fetal Research

Wm Daniel Cobb

The Ethics
of
Fetal Research

Paul Ramsey

New Haven and London
Yale University Press 1975

Designed by Sally Sullivan
and set in Times Roman type.
Printed in the United States of America by
Alpine Press Inc., South Braintree, Mass.

Published in Great Britain, Europe, and Africa by
Yale University Press, Ltd., London.
Distributed in Latin America by Kaiman & Polon,
Inc., New York City; in Australasia and Southeast
Asia by John Wiley & Sons Australasia Pty. Ltd.,
Sydney; in India by UBS Publishers' Distributors Pvt.,
Ltd., Delhi; in Japan by John Weatherhill, Inc., Tokyo.

To my grandson
Erik Marcus Ramsey

Contents

Introduction

We who are not scientists can begin to understand the nature and purposes of experiments using live human fetuses by classifying what is done or may be done into three sorts or types of research. In one type, the human research subject is the fetus in utero (most frequently, in anticipation of abortion). In another type, the subject is the still-living, previable abortus, the product of spontaneous or induced abortion, after it is disconnected from the placenta. A third type falls temporally between these two: in cases of abortion by hysterotomy (a procedure which emulates a Caesarian section), the fetus may be exteriorized, leaving its placenta in place, and then experiments may be conducted while it is still connected with the mother—before the umbilical cord is cut.

Examples of the sorts of research that can be done using the live human fetus at these times will fill in that sketch. In the last-mentioned case, for example, while the fetus is still connected with the mother, tests can be performed to determine whether a substance or substances pass from maternal circulation across the placental barrier into fetal circulation. This might be done by injecting a substance into the woman and at five-minute intervals taking samples of fetal blood. Fetal organs subsequently can be tested to determine whether the substance has lodged in them. Or a series of injections could be begun shortly before hysterotomy, continued while the procedure was being performed, and completed with the fetus exteriorized and still linked with the placenta.

Research using the still-living, previable abortus, separated from its mother, is usually directed toward developing improved ways of saving immature fetuses, or improving incubators for immature and premature neonates or infants. The goal is to save future human lives. Such attempted "salvage" or "rescue" techniques are the perfusion incubator and submergence in saline solution under hyperbaric pressure. In the first case a vein and an artery are cannulated, and the fetal blood is thus externally oxygenated and then circulated.

In the second case, the goal is to force oxygen through the skin. In both cases, the life of the previable abortus is experimentally extended, in the hope of learning how to save future babies until their lungs can expand and function. I suppose also that useful information might be derived from procedures that would of themselves directly kill or hasten the abortus' dying.

Research on the fetus in utero may consist of tests to determine whether given substances pass the placental barrier and harm the fetus; they may try to determine which are most efficient in giving aid and protection to the fetus. An example of the latter is the experiment (discussed below) to determine which of two antibiotics should be used instead of penicillin to treat in utero syphilis in the fetuses of women with penicillin allergies. An example of the former can be construed by imagining that thalidomide had been tested before it was allowed to be prescribed and marketed. Thalidomide, I understand, is quite a good drug for its purposes. However, it had tragic consequences for the children of women who used it in early pregnancy. These are some of the benefits to come and detriments to prevent by knowledge gained by experiments on the human fetus in situ, in anticipation of abortion. Indeed, in this pharmacological age, when at least everyone seeks to be discomfort-free, it can be claimed that all drugs, before they are marketed, ought to be tried on pregnant women who are planning an abortion! This would help to avoid future thalidomides.

This case does suggest, however, that there might be other ways to avoid some of the avoidable drug-induced damage to infants, namely by not prescribing so many drugs during pregnancy. Such other ways to limit the damage would need to be adopted if, as is the rule in Great Britain, sound medical ethics should prohibit medical research from administering drugs (or carrying out any procedure on the mother) with the deliberate intent of ascertaining the harm that these might do to the fetus.

Similarly, efforts to improve our techniques for saving the lives of babies born too immature to breathe, or to breathe well, need not come to a grinding halt if a sound medical ethics should conclude that such an advancement in medical science ought always to be connected with efforts to promote the lives of fetus/neonates who are on the borderline of viability, or just short of it. That would be the ethics of it, if we thought that the previable, but not yet dead, abortus ought not to be submitted (with deliberate intent) to certain damage in order to develop salvage techniques for other babies.

In the pages to follow I ask the reader to ponder the skewing of the ordinary canons of medical ethics when the fact of abortion is brought in to justify research using abortuses that are not yet dead. Not only do questions arise about how long—e.g. indefinitely?—it is morally permissible to sustain the life of an abortus for experimental purposes. More crucial and puzzling is the fact that ordinarily, "experimental treatment" seems far easier to justify ethically than research having no connection with therapy. Precisely that judgment is reversed in the case of the fetal research subject.

Experimentation on the fetus in utero, however, is by no means limited to drug studies. Ultrasound is or can soon be used in the early detection of fetal heart defects; such diagnosis can be important for treatment at birth. Physicians do not believe that the use of ultrasound is really damaging to the fetus. They would simply like to use the fetus in utero in anticipation of abortion to "prove" that this is the case, before bringing the diagnostic procedure into general use. Similarly, one of the researchers in the antibiotic experiment is quoted as saying, "There was no reason to think that either antibiotic would be harmful to a fetus—each is widely used—but it seemed wrong to take any chance."[1]

Then, ought we to understand ultrasound and antibiotic research to be rather like "controlled observation" of the fetus in utero and commend it? Or like my construed thalidomide experiment, as seeking to determine the harm to the fetus, and morally condemn it? These are some of the issues with which we wrestle in this volume.

Notice that in thus delineating the kinds of things that can be done in fetal research, with some examples, I have not said a word about the use of the dead fetus (whole and intact), or about the placenta (which is the fetus' "organ"), or about fetal tissue in research, or about fetal organs for transplants. Questions arising in these connections fall under the heading of our use of dead bodies, or at most our treatment of the newly dead. Their answers should be governed by regulations flowing from different principles and precautions: these are not at issue here.

Two things, however, should be pointed out in this connection. First, both the foes and the proponents of abortion frequently confuse research using fetal tissue or the dead abortus with research using the human fetus in situ or the previable living abortus—the one to escalate its moral outrageousness, the other to praise its great and indispensible benefits. Both poison the wells of public-policy formulation in the matter of fetal research.

Second, the important information that can be gained from simply using the dead fetus, the placenta, and fetal tissue is often not fully taken into account. If there are reasons for protecting the fetal human subject in research, or even if we only ought never do research on the live fetus unless the information is highly significant and can be procured by no other means, the possibilities of potentially beneficial research on fetal tissue even if at greater cost and delay need to be fully explored. In discussing such issues, some scientists I have heard say, "You don't need to do fetal research in order to learn *that*." The public needs to know more about that statement—and in detail—if we are to be sufficiently informed to make sound judgments about how we want medical progress to be made.

Certain borderline problems may arise in limiting fetal research, while permitting fetal-tissue research. A prohibition of nonbeneficial research on the living abortus, I am told, could impede enzymatic and viral investigations, which depend on fresh skin fibroblasts. There are enzyme deficiencies and viral infections that can be properly studied only in fresh cells. That means that if the definition of death of the fetus entails a risk of prolonged underperfusion of skin, such studies could become rare. Then the question is whether a proper declaration of fetal death need impede this sort of investigation.

I grant the benefits to be obtained from fetal research—

especially if "obtained as rapidly as possible" or in a less roundabout or costly manner stands unchallenged as among the "benefits." It is for the scientists—not the ethicist—to tell us all we need to know about the medical benefits at issue, and also, in far more specific detail, about the nature of fetal research procedures. For our purposes in discussing the ethics of fetal research, the above typology will suffice.

My examples, however, are not nearly sufficient to indicate fully why researchers want to do fetal research. Broadly speaking, they believe that progress in fetal physiology, our knowledge of prenatal development, and many benefits to come in the practice of fetal medicine are at stake. Especially crucial are future possible treatments of genetic defects in utero.

The broadest area of need is for data on normal fetal development, not just in gross morphology but at the level of cellular and subcellular function. If therapeutic interventions in inborn errors of metabolism are ever to be applied to affected fetuses, so that they can be treated in utero rather than aborted, an enormous amount of groundwork involving data on normal fetuses at various stages will be needed. This is necessary for increasing understanding of why birth defects occur, as a prerequisite for prevention, and as a baseline for possible genetic therapy of fetuses afflicted with inborn errors of metabolism, so that they might be treated in utero rather than face the alternatives of abortion or birth in a handicapped state. Interpretation of possible intervention research is impossible, I am told, without data on normal fetuses.

Some interesting progress in early intervention in birth defects in lower vertebrates suggests that human applications might be considered in the foreseeable future. Some of this will require greater skill in early detection of defects, using ultrasound, fetoscopy, and the like. There is recent progress in intrauterine detection of congenital heart malformations by ultrasound, which would allow the mother to deliver in a high-risk perinatal unit, where the affected infant can receive life-saving treatment, rather than risk neonatal death consequent to being born in a nursery incapable of dealing with the problem. Again I understand that further refinements in using ultrasound require data on normal fetuses.

One of the most important areas of recent research relates to the prevention of hyaline membrane disease (a major cause of death and disability in premature infants) by prenatal assessment of lung maturity, so that decisions regarding the optimal time for delivery can be based on reliable data, and for the purpose of treating fetuses with immature lungs with corticosteroids, which seem to stimulate the enzyme necessary for production of the substance which prevents hyaline membrane disease. Such investigations require amniocentesis (the prenatal monitoring of normals), with all the risks of that procedure, and could be done more reliably if more were known of the possible adverse effects of corticosteroids on midtrimester fetuses. That could be learned with pre-abortion fetuses.

Other areas of inquiry which might be threatened by drawing certain sorts of lines on fetal research include intrauterine treatment of intrauterine infections, a major cause of birth defects and mental retardation; intervention in early embryogenesis to correct maldevelopment; development of an artificial placenta; hybridization in the fertilized egg to correct enzymatic deficiencies; and an enormous area of investigation involving effects of maternal attitudes and affect on the fetus and child-to-be. All of these areas are at a stage where beneficial applications within the foreseeable future are reasonably to be expected. They all involve questions which can be more reliably answered by studies which would initially involve non-beneficial interventions.

Some of the possible "fetal" research would technically be embryo research, involving experiments which could be done on conceptuses less than eight weeks old, in anticipation of abortion prior to eight weeks, but this would obviously come to involve true fetuses, by delay of abortion until after eight weeks in some instances. The upshot of such research might ultimately lead to therapeutic interventions at the embryo stage with the intent of promoting the development of a healthy fetus. In this instance, certainly, serious question would be raised about the ethics of the experimental procedure because it involves altering the time of the abortion for experimental purposes. Should that be done to the developing fetus and to pregnant women even with their consent?

These are some of the things I have gleaned from physician-researchers. I trust I have given a fairly accurate statement of their best cases. It is puzzling to me that some medical men who have chosen to speak out on this issue have selected weaker cases—especially research findings that can be procured by other means. If I do not misunderstand them, some defenders want to do fetal research just because it is there as a possibility, or because it might more rapidly advance medical science, or simply because they want to be free from the ethics that a wider human community might impose.

There is both a *how* and a *whither* in the total case for or against fetal research: means and ends are involved. In this volume I grant the medical benefits to come. On that point, a moralist might have some important observations concerning some of the *social* and *moral* prices unavoidably linked with the medical benefits: for example, the corruption or hardening of the lifesaving and healing professions and the skewing of medical ethics if we simply seize the "golden opportunity" afforded by the widespread practice of abortion. An ethicist must insist, in season and out of season, that the moral history of mankind is more important than its medical history. In addition, some of the interventions mentioned above, which aim to develop prenatal treatments and to save premature babies, will lead inevitably to the possibility of complete extracorporeal gestation and to gene change of every sort. That means that among the results we face are the manufacture of the children of future generations and growing them in vitro. The proximate results may be beneficial, while the ultimate result may be Aldous Huxley's hatchery. Anyone who thinks seriously about the morality of fetal research, then, should sort out the "benefits" and count the costs.

But that is not all. Today one often hears statements like, "fetal research must be done," or "it would be immoral not to do this research." The validity of such opinions and utterances entirely depends on a net-benefits ethics. It is a moralist's business to reply that there are more right-making and wrong-making ingredients in ethical analysis and judgment than beneficial consequences; there are other moral imperatives besides "the research imperative." To make this reply would require a full-scale ethical argument, or rather an argument about the nature of ethical reasoning and ethical "concluding," which I do not undertake here. Suffice it is to say that an immediate, untroubled, and uncomplicated justification of fetal research is thoughtless—because it assumes something that is questionable in ethics—the correctness of a net-benefits ethics, and that only.

My discussion of the ethics of fetal research must be set within the context of the existing standards of medical ethics. These are not net-benefits ethics alone; such is not the meaning of "do no harm." Nor are the ordinary canons of medical ethics—its permissions and its abstentions—simply an elaboration of the second article of the Nuremberg Code, "the experiment should be such as to yield fruitful results for the good of society, unprocurable by other methods or means of study, and not random and unnecessary in nature." Standing alone, that might permit cruelty, harm, injury or pain—provided they are not inflicted randomly, wantonly, or without good design.

For this reason, I begin, continue, and end this book with the various efforts in the early 1970s to formulate guidelines permitting fetal research in the United States and Great Britain. Not one of these assumes a net-benefits ethics alone or presupposes that the only moral norm or warrant is that research be "unprocurable by other methods or means of study." We must do some hard thinking about abortus research, if in the days ahead medical ethics is not to be "aborted" or at least severely damaged by the trauma of ill-considered debate over the use of the human fetus in medical experimentation.

In the course of this small volume, my own opinions are clear enough. But I would sooner have answers to my arguments than attention to my conclusions. I fancy myself engaged in the pursuit of "the truth to be done." This undertaking tries to raise the level of the current debate: at a time when persuasive appeals, heightened emotional utterances, non sequiturs, and opinions plainly dangerous to the moral becoming of humankind have served as surrogates for "good reasons." I am not sure that I quite live up to the standard set by the description of this volume: "The reader is not told what to think about research on human fetuses, but how to think about this new form of human research." Still this is, at least, my aim.

Consider the following standards that entail drawing different lines on fetal and abortus research:

1. A medical practitioner may/may not/carry out procedures on the mother with the deliberate intent of ascertaining the *harm* that these might do to the fetus.

2. A medical practitioner may/may not/carry out procedures on the mother with the deliberate intent of ascertaining the *benefit* these might do to the fetus, where abortion is in prospect and the fetal research subject itself will not benefit.

3. A medical practitioner may/may not/carry out procedures on the mother or with a previable abortus that entail *discernible risk* of harm to the fetus.

4. A medical practitioner may/may not/ . . . unless they entail *discernibly no risk* . . .

5. . . . unless there is no conceivable risk . . .

6. A medical practitioner may not *use* the fetus or abortus or neonate as a means (only) in research entirely directed to the benefit of others and not even remotely to its own medical benefit.

These optional regulations point to a range of objective and subjective morally relevant considerations. There is, first, the distinction between the intent to ascertain harm and the intent to ascertain benefit. However, even if there is intent to ascertain benefit, some of the foregoing optional regulations refer for final verdict to whether there is objectively "no discernible risk," "discernibly no risk," or "no conceivable risk" to the human fetal research subject from the proposed research protocol. Which shall be the measure—intention to harm, or risk of harm? Do we judge all attempts at determining the degree of benefit to the fetus to do no harm to the fetal subject because of the intention of the researchers? Or instead, are medical experimental investigations to be appraised (apart from the researcher's intent to ascertain benefit) in terms of whether the experimental intervention entails "no discernible risk," or (a more rigorous test) "discernibly no risk," or (stronger still) "no conceivable risk," or "no use as a means" (this Kantian standard puts all balancing benefit-judgments out of commission)? Is the objective to protect fetal human subjects from risk of harm, or from being used while in no way treated; from battery, or from being made the unknowing means in the acquirement of useful knowledge? (At law, of course, an "unconsented touching" is an assault and battery, and not only a harmful touching.) On the continuum between harm and no conceivable risk, which (if any) of these optional regulations should be deemed the equivalent to "controlled observation," or merely "systematic or pre-planned study" of the fetus? Which is perfectly harmless and arguably not an objectionable use of the fetus: No conceivable risk? Discernibly no risk? Is that also true of procedures having no discernible risk, or none (yet) discerned? Are only the discernible or discerned risks of imposed procedures morally impermissible? How "negligible" must the possible scientific risks be for them to be morally negligible? Finally, what is the research value of interventions that introduce so little risk that the experiment can morally be performed? Do not the research gains decrease as the risk of harm approaches the equivalence of systematic observation (a use that arguably is no abuse)?

There is a nest of unresolved issues here. Until they are resolved and a standard made clear, fetal research would entail treating similar experimental subjects dissimilarly, e.g. in terms of the harm permitted in research in different medical centers. That would be a species of unfairness or injustice.

The remarkable fact is that the framers of the proposed American guidelines are extraordinarily unwilling to go further in refining the regulations in any of the ways suggested by these options. Instead, as we shall see, the first "notice," or provisional draft, that was published categorically prohibited research on the fetus in utero in anticipation of abortion—because medicine's duty to do no harm was in no way weakened by planned abortion or a woman's consent—while the revision published only months later allowed (it would seem) almost any experimentation, so long as it was simply a part of an abortion procedure. The justification for that appears to be the odd principle that two harms or wrongs (or one harm, and one legality) make a right, so long as the two are coincident in time.

The effort to keep the determination of risk or harm within the discretion of the researcher, peer committees, or "exceptions" allowed by the Secretary of Health, Education, and Welfare (if the risk is small) is of a piece with the reluctance of the framers of the proposed American guidelines to use gram weight, gestational age, and length from heel or rump to crown to define pre-viability on the safe side in determining the fetus' eligibility to be made a research subject. By "defining pre-viability on the safe side," I mean taking into account (1) a physician's possible subjective error in estimating gestational age: he may be a month off; and (2) the objective fact that, at any stage of medical science, there is not a line but a span of "possible viability" in between a certainly nonviable fetus and a certainly viable one. Surely we do not mean to do experimentation on possibly viable fetuses.

The medical research profession is going to have to be more open than heretofore on so urgent an issue. In the matter of fetal research in particular, and human experimentation generally, medical practitioners need not only to do right but today they must be seen to do right.

It still must be said that the guideline-drawing has gone a long way toward defining this somewhat novel research subject, the human fetus or abortus. We are approaching a conceptual definition of the "fetal human being," not only in terms of the pre-viability requirement but also in terms of its vital signs earlier in life, and in terms of what may or may not be done to that living human subject.

Therefore it is in order for me to speak occasionally of the "fetal human being." I do not say "person." There is a need for a more neutral expression, a word less laden with controversy. Perhaps "fetal human life" would do as well. If any reader feels that "being" connotes the same as "person," simply substitute "fetal human subject": the guidelines we are to examine are entitled "Protection of Human Subjects," and the human fetus is located among all other subjects needing protection in human experimentation. Certainly, "embryo," "fetus," "neonate," even "newborn" are terms of art, words we learn to use and impose, for certain important practical purposes, on the continuum of human development. They summarize a cluster of medical needs and medical practice. Moreover, always to say "fetus" in discussing the ethics of fetal research is as question-begging and laden with moral controversy as to insist on always saying "person." So I suggest that "embryonic human being," "fetal human being," "abortus human being," "neonatal or newborn human being" grasp rather well the reality we are to talk about, precisely because the stage of development is properly placed in an adjectival, not substantive, position. We understand that to be the case when we say "an adult" in referring to a member of that class of human beings. If a reader means by a "human being" a "person," I suggest that he occasionally try instead "embryonic human subject," "fetal human subject," "abortus human subject," or "neonatal human subject." These are a little ponderous, perhaps, but still less controversy laden than "person"—or "fetus," when used in ethical reasoning and not in strictly scientific contexts.

That can stand as the opening of our discussion of "the ethics of fetal research." There is another theme, an equally important one, and also an ethical matter: fetal research and public policy. Chapter 1 plunges immediately into the issue, and throughout the volume the running account of the events and processes by which various formulations of American guidelines or proposed policies came into being make the issue vividly clear. Medical-policy formulation raises the same question as public-policy formulation in all other areas: how, in a representative democracy do we—through the courts, administrative agencies, national commissions or Congress—insure that the public has a voice and that the moral judgments of a wider human community gain their proper influence in setting medical research policy? My view is that we, the people, are the final authority within constitutional limits in determining how in future we mean to be healed—when the means is human experimentation. The technical expertise of the medical research community cannot be the sole or chief arbiter in this matter, which is a question of morality and public policy. We have not yet found the decision-making procedures from which we can confidently expect ethical and political wisdom.

Thanks again are due to Doris (Mrs. Joel) Nystrom for the typescript, to my editor at the Yale University Press, Jane Isay, and to a number of physicians, ethicists, and lawyers with whom I have discussed the medical, ethical, and legal aspects of fetal research. They shall remain nameless because there are so many. However, I am especially grateful to LeRoy Walters for his pioneering article on the ethics of fetal research, to which I make several references below.

Some of the analysis set down in these pages was first worked out for a Workshop on Medical Ethics, sponsored by the Institute of Society, Ethics, and the Life Sciences, Hastings-on-Hudson, New York; and I am grateful to Dr. Robert M. Veatch of the Institute staff for the invitation to speak to that interdisciplinary group.

May the one to whom this little volume is dedicated grow up to understand some of the things for which his grandfather stood in his time and place.

Princeton University
Princeton, New Jersey
December 1974

PAUL RAMSEY

Chapter 1

Background History and Guidelines

THE BRITISH GUIDELINES

While medical experimentation on the human fetus is not exactly a new occurrence, discussion of fetal research as an issue in medical ethics is of relatively recent origin. The human fetus is, therefore, a novel subject of investigation in medical ethics, and the discussion has in fact hardly begun.

The public debate began in Great Britain, and was shortly concluded there, before the subject came to public attention in the United States. While God so loved the world that he did not send a committee, one is sometimes necessary in the governance of human affairs. So it came to pass that when Norman St. John-Stevas, M.P., gave prominence to reports of the commercial sale of human fetuses for research purposes in Great Britain in a speech to Parliament, an advisory group was appointed to draw up regulations, chaired by Sir John Peel, Fellow of the Royal College of Obstetrics and Gynecology. In May 1972 the report of the advisory group, on "The Use of Fetuses and Fetal Material for Research" was issued.[1] (It is also par for government-by-consensus commissions that St. John-Stevas was not a member of the advisory group.)

While the Peel Report is an admirable document, I cannot agree with G. R. Dunstan's judgment that "the matter proved to present no major ethical difficulty"[2] or that there remain no unresolved moral questions to be addressed to the British code of practice.

It is difficult to understand why Dunstan believes the Peel Report laid to rest all the ethical issues, since he himself seeks a point in human development "presumably related to the neural development of the fetus, at which the fetus becomes *relationally* dependent on its mother . . . [when] her *presence* to the fetus begin[s] to awaken in the fetus the potential of human response . . ." Such a point would be "a threshold at which experiment must cease, a step which must not be crossed. For beyond it lies the life of a man, the image and glory of God: and this is holy ground."[3] Dunstan follows Bernard Häring in locating relational humanity from the development of the cerebral cortex, which he says is from about the fortieth day.[4] Since the Peel Report allows experiments up to 20 weeks or 140 days, Dunstan should have ethical difficulties with that document.

The Peel Report used instead the safe side of viability to define a class of fetal human beings eligible for use in research. It stated that a fetus of over gestational age 20 weeks would be regarded as viable for purposes of research policy. That is to say, any experiment on a fetus viable as so defined was prohibited unless consistent with treatment necessary to promote its life. Within the foregoing definition of viability, experimentation on the whole "pre-viable" fetus was permissible only if also it weighs less than 300 grams (less than ¾ pound, lower than the weight-standard in the first U.S. proposals which would have allowed research to go up to 500 grams, or 1.1 pounds). The Peel Report found supporting evidence for its line-drawing in the fact that "in the pre-viable fetus of 300 grammes or less as distinct from the fetus approaching full term those parts of the brain on which consciousness depends are, as yet, very poorly developed structurally and show no signs of electrical activity." The last statement is a glaring scientific error, since electrical activity of the fetal brain has been monitored very much earlier; and, of course, in any comparison of the 300-gram fetus with near full term or with an infant, there is a continuum from poor to more complete structural development of the cortical regions of the brain.

In addition to describing this new class of human research subject on the safe side of viability, the British guidelines also distinguish the previable fetus from a dead fetus: the new subject of experimentation shows "some but not all signs of life."

The Peel rules require also that "the intending research worker" have no part in deciding a fetus' eligibility for experimentation; that it be shown that "the required information cannot be obtained in any other way," that no procedures be carried out during pregnancy "with the deliberate intent of ascertaining the harm that they might do to the fetus"; and that there be no monetary exchange for fetuses or fetal material, except enough to "meet the necessary costs incurred in administering those services."

The account given of the criminal law in Great Britain is that "the protection afforded to the fetus is continuous and is not abrogated by the fact that it may be the intention at the time of the infliction of the injury that the fetus should be prevented by a subsequent abortion from attaining life." Parallel to that interpretation of the criminal law, the Peel Report states,

> in our view it is unethical for a medical practitioner to administer drugs or carry out any procedures on the mother with the deliberate intent of ascertaining the harm that these might do to the fetus, notwithstanding that arrangements may have been made to terminate the pregnancy and even if the mother is willing to consent to such an experiment.

Concerning the abortus delivered alive, the report states, "in our view when the fetus is viable after delivery the ethical obligation is to sustain its life so far as possible and it is both unethical and illegal to carry out any experiments on it which are inconsistent with the treatment necessary to promote its life."[5]

Other provisions of the advisory group will be introduced in the discussion to follow.

THE FIRST AMERICAN ATTEMPTS
TO FORMULATE FETAL RESEARCH POLICY

The course of events in the United States was characteristically more tumultuous. Early in 1973, a doctors' newspaper, *Ob-Gyn News,* published documents that originated separately and had been for some time under consideration in the advisory council and in the Human Embryology and Development Study Section of the National Institute of Child Health and Human Development (NICHD). A "study section" is charged with providing the scientific review of research proposals to a National Institute of Health (NIH), while an "advisory council" determines the importance or public priority to be assigned specific proposals in dispensing federal funds. The latter also advises on the general policies of the NIH. A study section draws its members from the scientific community and is appointed by the institute's director. An advisory council has among its members representatives of the public, and it is appointed by the Secretary of Health, Education, and Welfare (HEW).

Both the advisory council and one study section of the NICHD had been preparing for more than a year statements on fetal research policy. Portions of all of these statements, together with excerpts from the ongoing discussion of those guidelines, were published by *Ob-Gyn News* (April 15, 1973). The *Washington Post* brought that (forthcoming) news article together with its own interviews with a number of prominent physicians and researchers to form a sensational story, published on April 10, 1973. The common belief for a time—and this includes participants in those deliberations—was that an insider had leaked the reports to *Ob-Gyn News*, hoping to prevent the issuance of policy decisions that he opposed. That is not what happened, but—if only to maintain suspense—let us look first at the substance of the American deliberations which came to light in April 1973. This consisted of the thinking developed in two different committees that had not worked in concert.

More than a year previous to the disclosure—as far back as March 1972—the advisory council to the NICHD had proposed regulations permitting fetal research. That document was comparatively bland: it urged that fetal research must go forward, under acceptable ethical and scientific guidelines; it applied to the fetus the provisions protecting the rights of minors and other helpless subjects; it required informed consent to be obtained from the appropriate party(ies); it charged review committees with insuring that the investigator not be involved in the decision to terminate a pregnancy, the "product" of which was intended for study within his own research. An observant reader would notice the additional charge that the rights of the mother and fetus be fully considered. It was not explained how the human fetus can be said still to be a bearer of "rights," or what rights remain, if the experiments are done when abortion is in view or has already been set on course.

At the same time another set of recommendations (dating from September 1971) was reported from the NICHD Human Embryology and Development Study Section. These were being debated by the advisory council. After the usual comments to the effect that planned scientific studies of the human fetus "must" be encouraged and that "acceptable" formats and safeguards "must" be found, those recommendations took a different tack. In agreement with the British commission, they used a series of descriptive statements on the safe side of viability to distinguish fetuses eligible for research from those that are not. They also distinguished "two distinct kinds of fetal subjects: the fetal patient—an undisturbed fetus in situ; the abortus—an isolated product of planned or spontaneous termination of pregnancy during the first 20 weeks of gestation." To the first, guidelines protecting the welfare of minors or other helpless subjects apply without modification. To the second, an isolated abortus, regulations should not differ from those governing research involving tissue or organs. Significantly, the report affirmed that "techniques for the temporary maintenance of functional integrity of isolated organs shall be applicable without further restriction for terminal studies of the [whole] abortus."

That left the Human Embryology and Development Study Section with a task of line-drawing, circumscribing the outer limits of a still "living" abortus eligible for research, in distinction from a fetus in situ or a premature infant. This it did by statements descriptive of the abortus on the safe side of viability. An "abortus" used in human experimentation, the report stated, "must meet at least two out of three criteria: it must be (1) no older than 20 weeks; (2) no more than 500 grams (1.1 pounds) in weight; and (3) no longer than 25 centimeters (9.8 inches) from crown to heel."[6] (The Peel Report, as we have seen, mentions no length, and draws the line on weight at 300 grams or ¾ pound).

To anticipate a conclusion to be reached later on from a

review of subsequent attempts to formulate American fetal research policy, it is of first importance that we now go back to
the beginning and reinstate one or another of these descriptions
of this new research subject *on the safe side of viability*.

Concerning fetuses or abortuses thus made eligible for medical experimentation, The *Washington Post* article commented,
in words that are applicable either to the British or to the U.S.
standards proposed in 1971 but disclosed in 1973: "Such tiny
infants if delivered intact may often live for an hour or so with
beating heart after abortion." While they cannot live longer
"unaided," because their lungs cannot be expanded or function,
they can be kept alive for three or four hours with the artificial
aid of fresh blood and oxygen otherwise administered.

One gathers from the *Post* account that the Human Embryology and Development Study Section, for some unstated reason, warned only that "under no circumstances should attempts
be made to keep a fetus [eligible in the foregoing terms] alive
indefinitely for research." (This, too, as we shall see, is a requirement that needs to be reinstated.) Meantime, the British
guidelines had been drawn up not only to end a scandal arising
from the commercial sale of fetuses to researchers but, the *Post*
said, also to end what "virtually everyone agreed was an abuse
—obtaining months-old fetuses for research and keeping them
alive for up to three or four days." While there is serious practical need for some such regulation if live abortus research is permitted, anyone who believes these are distinctions having final
moral significance must also believe that length of time span—
three or four hours, three or four days, or indefinitely—can
change the quality or the "moral species" of a human action or
a medical practice.

From NIH came prompt denials that either report was "at
the present time policy," as Dr. Charles U. Lowe, scientific
director of NICHD, put it; the reports had "no standing except
as a council expression." Of course, strictly speaking, nothing
a council says is policy; it is only an advisory body. But its influence was not denied. Because of the articulate Catholic
minority in the U.S., Dr. Lowe went on to say, and an articulate
Black minority sensitive on issues of human life and "genocide,"
it is doubtful that we should "go along with Great Britain, using

federal dollars" for fetal research. The NICHD was supporting no research using "live, intact fetuses," he said; to say whether *any* NIH institute was doing so would require a close survey of 12,000 projects.

Members of the staffs of certain senators say that in the weeks that followed it was reluctantly conceded to them that "a few," then "a lot" of fetal research projects were being funded. That situation is to be understood as follows. The NIH does fund "training grants" to medical centers here and abroad; the grantee need state only the training given. Therefore, there could be fetal research indirectly and unknowingly funded by NIH, provided the funds for that sort of research itself comes from other sources than federal tax dollars.

Part of the sensationalism of the *Post* article was provided by the remarks of Dr. Kurt Hirschhorn of New York's Mt. Sinai Hospital and Medical School; and the question remaining in public consciousness was whether some of the viewpoints he expressed are not, in fact, the rationale behind more carefully expressed defenses of fetal research. "How do we know what drugs do to the fetus unless we find out?" he asked. He seemed to associate himself with the opinion of those who say, We're not doing any harm to a fetus that's going to die anyway; we need to learn more about cells in the differentiation of organs in the body; we need to learn more about inborn anomalies. Since "it is not possible to make this fetus into a child," Hirschhorn concluded, "*therefore* we can consider it as nothing more than a piece of tissue" (italics added). As Dr. D. T. Chalkley, chief of the NIH Institutional Relations Branch said, "The determination of what research can be . . . acceptable depends on the *salvageability* of the fetus. . . . If you have a clearly nonviable fetus you are in a position to . . . possibly . . . treat it as nonviable tissue."[7] Prospective viability was the only characteristic of humanness or sign of life to be respected in the unborn. Unlike the Peel Report, Chalkley did not define the eligible fetus on the safe side of salvageability, nor did he mention the other signs of life that distinguish this human research subject from a dead fetus or fetal tissue.

On this view, there would then be no need for any ethical guidelines or limitations on fetal research except the determination of viability. Dr. André Hellegers, professor of obstetrics and director of the Kennedy Institute for the Study of Human Reproduction and Bioethics, Georgetown University, made a strong reply: that means "we want to make the [lack of] chance of survival the reason for the experiment. . . . If it's going to die, you might as well use it." If that is not "the British approach [as it, standing so *alone,* was not], it was certainly," Hellegers observed, "that of the Nazi doctors."[8]

What happened then, and what was said by responsible officials at NIH following the reports in April 1973 of plans and permissive guidelines for fetal research that had been in preparation for more than a year?

Not only was there some considerable public dismay and outcry, but a protest was organized by senior girls at the Stone Ridge Country Day School of the Sacred Heart in Bethesda, Md., adjacent to the NIH, joined by marchers from Landon Boys School (Protestant). (The participation of Protestant and other young people among the protesters was never mentioned in the news reports. Here was a small beginning of the anti-Catholic politization of the issue.) That, I suppose, was about to mushroom onto the 7 o'clock news on television, by which we Americans customarily make policy.

Whereupon, Dr. Robert Berliner, deputy director for science at the National Institutes of Health, called the protesters in and read to them (and on that occasion also to the American public) a sweeping denial. "The NIH does not now support research on live aborted human fetuses," he said, "and does not contemplate approving the support of such research. We know of no circumstances at present or in the foreseeable future which would justify NIH support of research on live aborted human fetuses." On that same occasion, Dr. John F. Sherman, acting director of the NIH, indicated that the official position of the NIH was substantially stronger than a simple decision to keep its funds from supporting such research. In addition, he affirmed that any NIH-supported scientist found to be doing experiments on live aborted fetuses (abroad or in the U.S., supported by private funds) would be asked to stop, even if the research was not being done with funds from the institutes (at pain of being denied funds for his other, acceptable research).[9]

That seemed a categorical ban. During the next seven months, the average informed member of the American public had every reason to believe that experimentation on whole, still-living fetuses was not and would not become accepted policy for national medical research. Such a concerned citizen had every reason to believe he could worry about something else, and that that would not be done in his name. When he made his announcement, Dr. Berliner assured the press and public that while his statement fell short of a formal NIH regulation, it would do as well; it had the support of Dr. John F. Sherman. "I don't think," he said, "there is any disagreement by anyone in the office of the director of NIH, so if I got run over by a truck tomorrow, it [the policy] would still stand."[10]

More than a truck was in preparation, or continued to be worked on after that episode. Subsequently Dr. Berliner's announcement was termed a "status" statement, not a "policy" statement. Nevertheless, when next the public could look in on fetal research policy formation seven months after these events, the product of the uninterrupted in camera deliberations of our research establishment had attained a higher level of rationality and moral acceptability than would have been the case had policy been frozen at the time of the *Ob-Gyn News* disclosures in April 1973, with the single exception that the definition of an eligible abortus on the safe side of viability was dropped.

What happened in April had not been a leak. It resulted from an inadvertance. Congress had passed the Freedom of Information Act, mandating that advisory counsels to all departments in the federal bureaucracy, including the NIH, must hold only open meetings. Times and places of their meetings had to be announced in the *Federal Register*. The members of the advisory council of NICHD whose deliberations were reported in *Ob-Gyn News* simply forgot that the act had gone into effect in 1973. The study section proposal was also before the council that day. A reporter from *Ob-Gyn News* was there with his tape recorder and was not recognized. The committee continued to talk as usual. That is how both proposals came to light. Then leaders of the medical research establishment spoke to quiet the storm: successful efforts they were.

THE ORIGIN OF "PROTECTION OF
HUMAN SUBJECTS" (1973)

Approximately seven months later, after a long silence in the public forum, a document entitled "Protection of Human Subjects: Policies and Procedures" (NIH proposed guidelines) was published in the *Federal Register*.[11] This was a notice of intention to recommend that the Secretary of Health, Education, and Welfare administratively promulgate these recommendations as guidelines governing human research in the United States. For the first time, two prior public notices were planned in the federal medical rule-making process. Interested parties were invited to submit written comment on the proposals. Normally, the *Federal Register* publishes once before promulgation by the secretary. This instance was unique because a preliminary draft was published. After the second notice, presumably, the process would terminate in a report promulgated by the secretary.

During this period Senator Edward Kennedy, D. Mass., was holding hearings on medical research and related questions, and among those who testified were members of the NICHD advisory council. The administrative branch invited only written comments. No public hearings were planned to stimulate public debate before the expected promulgation.

The document itself, however, provided for public participation in the administration of the regulations to an extent never before sought in medical research in the United States. If applying the rules ought to be *res publica,* we may ask why were the revision and the adoption of the rules so reserved to the medical community and not also conceded to be the public's business?

This is a basic question concerning medical policy formation. If research ethics should reflect the ethics of a wider human community, we need open covenants more openly arrived at. As we shall see, however, policy coming from the research community was interrupted—also an important occasion in our history—by the intervention of Congress.

Before turning to that other source of medical research rule-making at the federal level, a further comment is in order concerning the origins of the document, "Protection of Human

Subjects," to my mind the finest product to date—whatever its defects—to come from our federal medical bureaucracies. All classes of human subjects of experimentation, including fetal human beings, are considered, and a (perhaps too complicated) review procedure is elaborated to insure that they are effectively protected. These regulations and limitations surrounding fetal research are the best we have (next to the Peel Report), better than the subsequent revision published in August 1974 (which we take up later) and better than guidelines that might have issued from the 1973 deliberations published in *Ob-Gyn News*—except for the definition of viability measurably on the safe side for research purposes, which was dropped. None of the policies we shall take up for discussion and for ethical analysis are as yet promulgated for the United States, because of events that intervened from the congressional side.

First, however, some further remarks are in order about the origins of the fetal research sections of the 1973 NIH proposals. These concern ethical quandaries about the processes we have so far devised for medical-policy formation as one type of public-policy formation in democratic societies. The problem is whether the public has voice, whether we should have voice, and how we are to have an effective voice in the formulation of policies by which we or our children are in future to be healed.

The November 1973 policy concerning fetal research is a marked improvement over what seemed in the making, according to the disclosures in April 1973. It probably could not have been produced without avoidance of the Freedom of Information Act. During that silent seven months, deliberations did proceed. Internal evidence gives this credence, and so does external evidence: physicians, theologians, ethicists, lawyers (a number of whom I know) participated in the process. Meetings continued. Was this a circumvention of the Act? Did it violate its spirit? Deliberations continued, despite the public disclaimers made by leaders of our medical research establishment in April 1973, denying that we have or would have a policy funding fetal research. Can we say of that whole course of events that the public was deceived although nobody lied?

What was done was quite legal. Consultants were assembled.

They did not meet as an advisory council to which the Freedom of Information Act applies. In fact they did not even meet as a "body" of consultants. They met as an aggregate of individuals who were engaged in conversation with Dr. Charles U. Lowe, at NIH, advising him about the problem, presumably also talking with one another. They had no vote as a body of advisors. Such a consultation of experts had not to be noticed and open. Thus a reporter from *Ob-Gyn News* could not possibly attend.

The "consultation" with Dr. Lowe concerned perfecting fetal research policy and took up several other points that came out in the 1973 NIH proposed guidelines. The "representatives" of the public in this group had no control, however, over the final outcome. Revision continued on the document within NIH after the consultants no longer met. Still it seems obvious that the ethics of a wider human community must have been voiced by the nonscientific participants. The contrasting document is the 1974 revision produced strictly within NIH, without public participation, which was made on the basis of written responses, mainly from grantees (an inferior statement).

My quandary is, I believe, our quandary in democratic societies. How shall medical policy be formulated and enacted in matters that obviously involve serious moral and social questions, as well as scientific or technical questions? Should that be done by a process that terminates in the Secretary of Health, Education, and Welfare, with no appeal and with little public voice in the production of the regulations; with openness only through written comments submitted after the proposals have been drafted and (I have said, gratefully) published twice before the promulgation that was planned?

Here we have a sort of Daniel Ellsberg, Pentagon Papers, problem. The case might also be compared with recent allegations that the Atomic Energy Commission has not been candid about its own experts' studies of the dangers in nuclear reactors and power plants. I myself am ambivalent about the course of events that followed the categorical denials of any intention to permit or sponsor fetal research by Drs. Berliner and Sherman on April 18, 1973, in part because I judge the resulting NIH proposals to be a better product than might have issued earlier. The proposed protection of fetal human research subjects may have been improved precisely *because* the Freedom of Information Act was circumvented. Would legislation by Congress likely be better? Or the decisions of a national commission?[12] The latter, if it errs, may have gathered such prestige that further intervention by the public through Congress could be forestalled, or the courts unduly influenced.

As an ethicist of principles (not of consequences only) it is discomforting to have to acknowledge a case in which questionable means or procedures produced good results. Still it may be a salutary test for those of us who do not believe that the ends justify the means to confront an instance in which the ends, are substantially choiceworthy, while the way to them was morally dubious. That I think is a proper analysis of the present state of fetal research policy formation in the United States.

I myself believe in the importance of confidentiality in the process of policy decisions in a representative democracy. Still I venture to say that a Harris poll of the leaders of our medical research community would show that a majority of them do not believe that major policy decisions in regard to foreign affairs should be made in secret in the White House, State Department, or Pentagon. Such a poll would likely indicate the belief that Ellsberg acted in the nation's interest. I know for a fact that my colleague ethicists, theologians and otherwise, and my lawyer friends, who held meetings with Dr. Lowe after the public had been assured that there were no plans to legitimate fetal research in the United States, would generally say that a fatal flaw in military and foreign policy formation in the United States, or by the AEC, in recent years has been that too much has gone on behind closed doors, and that Ellsberg did the right thing by bringing military deliberations into the open. I know this because I have frequently half-jokingly told some of them that if they would only carry a tape recorder into one of those one-on-one meetings at NIH, I would gladly be the Dr. Ellsberg of the medical establishment.

I conclude from these speculations that the leaders of our medical research community should absorb the fact that many,

many Americans regard medical research policy decisions to be as important for our public morality as foreign affairs. In all areas the wisdom and rightfulness of public policies prepared beyond our reach depends upon genuinely enlisting the people's check, amendment, or rejection of those policies.

More than written comments should have been invited to the NIH guidelines; public hearings ought to have been held, ample time allowed, and positive efforts made to arouse public participation in a full-scale debate over national medical research policy. In this process, those who first formulated these proposals and other research physicians ought not—while participating as citizens—to "pull rank" or claim privileged expertise, as I think happens when dicta descend to the effect that research "must" be done on whole, still living abortuses. There's always an "if" attached to that; it is only a "conditional imperative." Anyone can understand the question whether we want rapid medical progress to be made—whether we want in future to be healed—by some or any means. The responsibility of the medical profession is simply to inform the public fully; even as, if fetal research is approved as public medical policy, they then ought fully to inform pregnant women about what exactly they propose to do and to learn. In both the public policy and the personal instances, the proposers of fetal research should await the answer; perhaps they should seek the answer they desire, but they should not try to fix it. As to the direction medical research should take for the remainder of this century, and particularly in regard to experimenting on condemned unborn fetal human beings, there is something to be said for André Hellegers' opinion: "Sometimes you have to take a vote *in order to get a minority opinion. . . .* I want to vote not in order to win or lose, but because I want my grandchildren to remember something about their grandfather." (italics added)[13]

Above I asked the question whether the formulation of public medical policy ought best to terminate in promulgations by the secretary of HEW. In 1974 the secretary issued regulations on another controversial moral and legal matter, sterilization. The fact that he did so emphasizes my questions both about the processes of policy formation and the final authority issuing policy.

During 1972 there were a number of news reports that uncomprehending minors were submitted to sterilization by agents administering federal family planning funds, and of a doctor in South Carolina who refused to deliver the babies of "welfare" mothers unless they agreed to tubal ligation. What happened then through the federal rule-making process terminating in the Secretary of Health, Education, and Welfare provides an interesting parallel to rule making in regard to the protection of human research subjects.

On August 3, 1973, DHEW published in the *Federal Register* a notice of "Guidelines for Sterilization Procedures under HEW Supported Programs," and on September 21, 1973, it published notice of detailed regulations for all agencies. Written comments were invited, and some 300 were received, including one from the National Welfare Rights Organization. The final regulations were promulgated by the secretary on February 6, 1974.

Undoubtedly, the secretary created a new class of permissible medical interventions (involuntary sterilization of minors and other incompetents and sterilization of welfare women inadequately protected from implied threat) under cover of regulating these practices. But in this instance there was recourse to the courts. The National Welfare Rights Organization brought suit to enjoin the use of federal funds for such purposes, and on March 15, 1974, Judge Gerhart A. Gesell of the U.S. District Court for the District of Columbia handed down an opinion ruling against the secretary, Casper W. Weinberger.[14] In this instance there was also an agreement of several interested parties: the American Civil Liberties Union and the U.S. Catholic Conference submitted *amicus curiae* briefs in support of the civil action brought by National Welfare Rights Organization.

The fact that the secretary was willing in the midst of a continuing storm of protests to promulgate regulations extending permission administratively to a new sort of medical intervention may be taken as a measure of the willingness of medical bureaucratic rule-makers to go against a more general public morality on behalf of their conception of a public health interest. Against the regulations, Judge Gesell declared: "Federally assisted family planning sterilizations are permissible only with the voluntary, knowing and uncoerced consent of individuals *competent to give consent"* (italics added). Even the dictionary definition of "voluntary," he said, "assumes an exercise of free will and clearly precludes the existence of coercion or force. . . . No person who is mentally incompetent can meet these standards, *nor can the consent of a representative,* however sufficient under state law, *impute voluntariness* to the individual actually undergoing irreversible sterilization. *Minors* would also lack the knowledge, maturity and judgment to satisfy these standards. . . ." (italics added)

Ordinarily there is not this immediate recourse to the courts, and decisions terminate in the secretary's office, if Congress does not intervene. On the matter of the protection of human research subjects, which is our chief concern here, James R. Nielsen, a lawyer on the faculty of the University of California Medical School and a member of its Committee on Human Experimentation has brought suit to enjoin experiments involving children in no need of treatment and on unconscious patients.[15] It is possible that a ruling as to law will be forthcoming from this case, which will demonstrate to medical researchers and administrators that the law is not really "unclear" or "confused" on these questions (they usually assert this, against the nearly unanimous opinion of lawyers). "Case law" is always uncertain and may change; more importantly, case law has no application unless someone can get standing to sue in civil or class-action cases. But that does not mean the law provides no clear guide.

With regard to medical research in general, there are likely to be few occasions afforded for resort to the courts. This is especially true in regard to protection of the fetal research subject. If administrative rule-making and the secretary's decrees are not to be and ought not to be autonomous, we should expect appeal to be made to state legislatures and further interventions from the Congress. "At a minimum," writes Gary L. Reback, a legal scholar who believes most of the state laws are poorly drawn, "American researchers should understand that they face a legislative ban on experimentation [on fetuses] unless a compromise solution is reached."[16]

CONGRESS ACTS

The NIH guidelines, "Protection of Human Subjects" was not promulgated for the following reasons. The delay of the secretary's promulgation for so many months might at the time have supported the suspicion that, on the matter of fetal research, the document was being weakened. However, the entire document is a complex one, and each complexity involves important medical, moral, and social issues. The revision took time. The fact was, however, that another source of possible federal medical rule-making intervened—the U.S. Congress— and cut across the rule-making originating from our health departments.

For some years there has been a public movement for a national commission created by the Congress to lead and oversee medical and scientific innovations that are of obvious overriding public concern. Senator Mondale, D. Minn., has been a leader of this drive. Yet despite diligent staff work, publicity, and congressional hearings under Mondale's leadership, no decision, even that we need a temporary commission to study and decide whether there is need for such a permanent commission or not, was reached.

But that situation has recently changed, and Congress may become an additional source of initial biomedical policy.

In July 1974 the Congress passed a National Research Act. Under Title III of that Act, "Protection of Human Subjects of Biomedical and Behavioral Research," a national commission with a life of only two years is to be appointed. It is expected to make recommendations concerning the functions and authority of a permanent National Advisory Council, which will be established on July 1, 1976. The commission's recommendations of provisions regulating research are to be published, and the secretary of HEW must publicly respond to each of them. If he rejects them, he must publish his reasons for doing so.

Among the specific tasks assigned the temporary commission is to make recommendations regarding fetal research and the use of psychosurgery—two issues that were in the news while this legislation was being formulated. The House bill had prohibited the secretary from conducting or supporting research on a human fetus which is outside of its mother and which has a beating heart. Senator James Buckley, R. N.Y., had proposed a similar prohibition in the Senate bill. Before passage Senator Kennedy proposed a "perfecting" amendment to the Buckley amendment, which had the effect of prohibiting fetal research only until the commission made its recommendations and the secretary responds or promulgates provisions relevant to that sort of human experimentation. That move also enabled senators and congressmen to pass the ball to the commission and avoided their having to take decisive stand on a controversial public question. Until that process is completed, the secretary is forbidden to conduct or support research or experimentation in the United States or abroad on a living human fetus, whether before or after induced abortion, unless such research is done for the purpose of assuring the survival of that fetus. It is mandated that the temporary commission shall make its recommendations on this issue (and psychosurgery) within four months after the date it comes into existence.

It is certainly a symbolic flaw, and a flaw of some practical consequences, that the Senate bill's reference to "whether before or after induced abortion" was in the final legislation. For it is only by the quantity of experimental subjects made available that there is significant linkage between current abortion practice and the moral issues involved in using living fetal human beings in medical experimentation. The product of a spontaneous miscarriage, if previable and not yet dead, places the same (or no) moral claims upon us.

The state of the question of fetal research at the Federal rule making level in the United States in July 1974 was the following. The paragraphs on that topic in the 1973 NIH "Protection of Human Subjects" policy proposal, together with written responses that may have been received and any further drafting done, would certainly be made a part of the commission's record, as it prepares to issue its recommendations four months into its two-year life. It may simply recommend something like those provisions. Or if it does not, the secretary of HEW still has the authority to reject its recommendation and for stated reasons to promulgate instead regulations like those already in preparation and about to emerge from the Federal bureaucratic process during 1974. Or he could state his reasons for promulgating quite different regulations.

One month after passage of the National Research Act, the secretary of HEW published in the *Federal Register*[17] a summary of responses to the November 1973 proposed guidelines and a revision of "Protection of Human Subjects"—"to continue the public dialogue," not as regulations in torce. These will be discussed below and in proper sequence.

The Secretary of Health, Education, and Welfare, Caspar W. Weinberger, on September 13, 1974, announced the selection of the eleven-member temporary national commission established by law to study and make recommendations for guidelines on the protection of human subjects.

Named to the commission were: Joseph V. Brady, Ph.D., professor of behavioral biology, School of Medicine, Johns Hopkins University; Robert E. Cooke, M.D., vice-chancellor for health and sciences, University of Wisconsin; Dorothy S. Height, president of the National Council of Negro Women, Inc.; the Rev. Albert R. Jonsen, S.J., Ph.D., adjunct associate professor of bioethics, School of Medicine, University of California; Patricia King, professor of law, Georgetown University Law Center; Karen A. Lebacqz, Ph.D., assistant professor of Christian ethics, Pacific School of Religion; David W. Louisell, J.D., professor of law, University of California, Berkeley; John Kenneth Ryan, M.D., chairman of the department of obstetrics and gynecology, Harvard University Medical School; Donald Wayne Seldin, M.D., professor and chairman of the department of internal medicine, University of Texas Southwestern Medical School; Eliot Stellar, Ph.D., provost of the university and professor of physiological psychology, University of Pennsylvania, and Robert H. Turtle, Esq., Washington, D.C.

The Commission was sworn in on December 2, 1974. Charged to report recommendations in four months on psychosurgery (where case law is an available recourse) and on fetal research (which case law ordinarily does not touch), these commissioners hold much of the future of medical ethics and research practice in their hands.

It is safe to say, however, that the moral and public policy questions in fetal research are not going to leave Congress alone, and the Congress is now unavoidably and deeply involved in these issues. The recommendations of the permanent National Advisory Council to come into being July 1, 1976, are expected to be disseminated to the public and to undergo extensive public discussion. The recommendations of the temporary commission or of the permanent National Advisory Council will still terminate in the secretary of HEW (who appoints them). Perhaps, then, policy will be made in much the same way as in the past if these bodies accumulate prestige enough to dampen congressional intervention.

On the other hand, the secretary has to state publicly his reasons if he does not agree with those recommendations. Members of congress may not be able to avoid making controversial points a matter of their legislative deliberations. Perhaps the question of fetal research will be addressed again in their solemn assemblies. That would mean that in camera determination of medical ethical issues is coming to an end, and the public is now deeply involved in debate over these questions. That may be a good thing—or not. For I have said in the course of this account that I, for one, expect no better rulings on fetal research to be put forth in the United States than those in the original NIH guidelines. That and the Peel Report will frame the systematic analysis of the ethical issues to follow.

Chapter 2
Types of Fetal Research

It may be worth briefly extending this anecdotal account of the emergence of fetal research as a medical-ethical question in the United States by recounting my own process of becoming aware of the issue.

The practice of several sorts of fetal research came to my attention some years before the whiplash of recent abortion doctrines greatly expanded its scope. For this reason it seemed obvious to me that in our late lamented abortion "debate" we were writing the agenda for another wrenching and fateful decision. This has to be pointed out, even though the ethics of abortion and the ethics of fetal experimentation are separate questions, as I will try to show. I was then writing on children in experiments and, so to speak, bumped into the other issue.

The experiments at George Washington University Hospital by Dr. Geoffrey Chamberlain on eight human fetuses ranging in weight from 300 to 980 grams, reported in 1968[1], first came to my attention. Because I was then interested in the protection of child-subjects, my eyes lighted upon the following instance of his investigations in trying to develop a rescue technique, the perfusion incubator (it is sometimes called artificial placenta):

A 14-year-old girl was admitted for termination of pregnancy. When the patient was seen, the uterus was at about 26 weeks' gestational size, and hysterotomy was performed. A 980-gram male fetus was delivered in his amniotic sac. Umbilical vein and both arteries were cannulated with no difficulty, about 11 minutes after separation of the placenta. Blood flowed evenly into the umbilical vein, but no return occurred from the arteries at first. However, brisk spontaneous flow occurred 22 minutes after birth and the fetus was established on the circuit; he stayed so for 5 hours, 8 minutes. The experiment stopped then because a cannula inadvertently slipped and could not be reintroduced.

Once the perfusion was stopped . . . the gasping respiratory efforts increased to 8 to 10 per minute. The fetus died 21 minutes after leaving the circuit.[1]

While that appeared to me to be a case of sustaining life in a previable abortus with the objective of developing an artificial placenta for future prematures, practicing physicians to whom I showed that description—to my astonishment—were unanimous in exclaiming that it was a viable baby. They went on to explain that taking the baby out in his sac meant in itself the researcher never intended to promote its survival. Some expressed scepticism about whether the cannula slipped "inadvertently."[2] Here too—as in a number of more recent cases of fetal research—some of the simple canons of experimentation ethics are sufficient to ground objection to what was done by Dr. Chamberlain. Is it credible to believe, for example, that that 14-year-old girl gave a valid consent? The researcher was nevertheless given a prize.

At a conference on experimental pharmacology, a representative of a pharmaceutical firm located in New Jersey told me that he was personally engaged in a research project that involved going to Japan and paying women planning abortions for permission to use fetus or abortus in drug studies.

My "intelligence" told me about a research protocol from Japan presented to NIH for funding. The objective was to study the speed of disposition of minerals into the fetal mandibles (jawbone). The protocol called for maintaining whole previable abortuses alive for up to three days, injecting the substance or substances being tested into the umbilical cord, and then at five-minute intervals cutting off the heads of a series of abortuses over the three day period in order to examine the jawbones of each at that point in time. I do not know how or what major vital signs were to be maintained, but evidently the jawbones and the abortuses as a whole were alive and well and growing, or else the protocol would have been pointless. The request was first approved and then, in a reversal, disapproved by an NIH "study section" which was charged with making the scientific review—reversed for the reason that the American public would not "understand" it.

Finally, I had brief correspondence with Dr. Robert C. Goodlin of Stanford University—brief because his interests were not then in the forefront of my concerns—who until 1969 was engaged in experiments using living, previable fetuses as subjects in trials of saline immersion plus hyperbaric oxygen as a potential approach to saving fetuses delivered with immature lungs. After 2,000 animal studies, his work was extended to 40 human fetuses that came from spontaneous or induced abortions, including hysterotomies. The longest he was able to keep a fetus alive was 11 days. Again, the experiments would have been pointless if those previable abortuses had not been importantly and relevantly "alive" before yet having capacity for respiration. Dr. Goodlin was recently reported to have said not only in regard to his 11-day wonder, "but with every one, I always insisted that this might be the fetus that makes it."[3] If Goodlin's research may be described as possibly, however remotely, beneficial to the experimental subject, his were therapeutic investigations, which are open to few objections—except that physicians should not begin useless or hopeless procedures if they are truly known or believed to be such, or procedures that may do more harm than help.

While this brief sketch of me and fetuses under experiments may be of only vanishing autobiographical significance, it does bring into focus several objectives of such research: the perfection of rescue techniques (by perfusion oxygenating and circulating the fetus until lungs are stronger, by oxygen under pressure in hope of forcing it through the skin), drug testing, the study of prenatal organ development; and the fact that some but not all such trials may be therapeutic. Let us, therefore, concede for the sake of focusing the moral argument that there are important benefits to other children to be derived from fetal research. The Peel Report's requirement that "the information cannot be obtained in any other way" would, indeed, eliminate some, perhaps a good deal, of the fetal research done today; but that requirement is surely met in many fetal studies.

Before taking up in the next chapter the sorts of moral considerations and arguments that are relevant, we ought to summarize descriptively the sorts of things that can be done in fetal studies into classifications of experimental procedures.

Fetal human beings are available as possible research subjects (1) in utero in the case of planned abortions. Here it will be said that risk of injury or pain to the fetus from the experimental procedure is clearly less serious than the death already decreed by an abortion decision, and therefore almost anything is allowable that promises beneficial medical information. To keep stressing—as today we must—that fetal experimentation is a separate issue from abortion, one might at this point refer to Dr. M. H. Pappworth's *Human Guinea Pigs*.[4] The early pages of that volume describe some rather astonishing imposition of risks upon the fetus in situ and upon pregnant women that was not done in anticipation of abortion. Undoubtedly, however, the wide practice of abortion has freed up experimental designs.

Fetal human beings are available as possible research subjects (2) as fetuses still connected by the umbilical cord to the placenta and to the mother's support system in cases of abortion by hysterotomy; and (3) as intact, still living abortuses after they are detached from the placenta and from maternal circulation (they may be spontaneously "born" before viability or produced by means of induced abortion—so long as they are produced alive).

Obviously, fetuses may be entered into research in some combination of these ways. Experimentation can begin on the subject in situ near the time of abortion and be completed by further tests while it is still attached to maternal circulation, or by blood tests or other studies following detachment. For this reason LeRoy Walters[5] distinguishes three types of fetal research according to the time span of the action: (1) experiments which begin at a significant time interval (one week or more) before intended abortion, (2) experiments begun shortly (several hours or days) before induced abortion, and (3) experiments begun only after the entire separation of fetus from mother. In Walters' example of Type (1), live rubella vaccine was administered during pregnancy to 35 women, and abortions were performed (and the study completed) between

11 and 30 days later.[6] In his example of Type (2) research intravenous infusions of ^{125}I-Glucagon were given to nine women several hours before abortion, followed by taking samples of maternal blood every 10 or 15 minutes and then of blood samples of the fetus after it "was exteriorized . . . while the fetus and mother were still attached and while the placenta remained intact in the uterus."[7]

To these types and examples should be added the use of fetal tissue for transplants to very young patients. A thymus gland taken from an abortus and implanted in a baby born without immunological competence can repair its lack of ability to resist infection and may save its life.

Whether the fetus is used as research subject or as organ donor, ethical questions are raised concerning the claims, if any, of the fetus, and what difference, if any, intended or actual abortion makes to the way fetuses should be treated. These issues I discuss in the pages that follow; and to do so, I analyse what is said in the two most recent American documents, the 1973 NIH-proposed guidelines and the 1974 DHEW-NIH revised guidelines, and the Peel Report in force in Great Britain.

Chapter 3
Themes in Ethical Analysis

While fetal research is something of a novelty in discussions of medical ethics, it would be a mistake to believe that it is unique, or to hold that there are no analogies to be drawn, no familiar settings in which to view the topic, or no guideposts to be found in our extant medical ethics for making a moral appraisal of this type of research. There are a number of themes or ingredients for medical ethical judgment that weave in and out, sometimes in such fashion that both apply and together are weighty, sometimes separating so that only one is the applicable criterion, or both may be but in such fashion that one alone suffices. Clear thinking requires that we be careful about the line or lines of moral reasoning we are using.

First, a decision has to be made whether fetal research is a species of human research, whether it is more like experimentation involving human subjects than "animal work." If it is more like research using live animals that like us are sensate creatures, researchers might be subject to many limitations deemed to be restrictions no less than if we class fetal with human research. By not addressing this and other questions about the applicable themes of medical ethics, and by leaving the matter in limbo, we would grant the freedom some spokesmen seem to desire, to design fetal research procedures by one test alone: beneficial knowledge to come.

The Peel Report takes up this question in response to the suggestion that licenses be issued to "those who wished to undertake research using fetuses, fetal tissue or fetal material similar to licenses issued to those undertaking research on animals." It replied: "In our view a system of licensing would be unnecessarily cumbersome and a code of ethical practice would be an adequate safeguard as it is in the case of research involving all patients." That was a backhanded way of saying clearly enough that the fetus is a *human* research subject.

27

Similarly, the very title "Protection of Human Subjects" in which U.S. policy makers discuss fetal research presupposes that this sort of experimentation is human, not animal investigation—and the word "subject" is at least as neutral as my occasional use of "being." The substance of the proposed guidelines also presuppose this to be the case. One does not protect tissue. Nor do we—if human benefits are seriously at stake—protect animals from more than pain and wanton wastage. The guidelines uniformly offer greater protection to the unborn, miscarried, or aborted human research subject (that is their point and not alone the mother and her feelings) than we do to animals.

It seems to me to be obvious that fetal research is human experimentation. Then a whole range of themes in research ethics become potentially applicable to the use of the fetal human being. We can sort some of them out by asking: To what else is the fetus to be likened?

The human fetus resembles the human embryo and the human infant more than anything else in creation; and of the two, it resembles a newborn infant more than it does an embryo.[1] If this is true, then a part of our task will be to ask: How do the standards governing children in nontherapeutic experimentation apply in this instance? Anyone who believes, for example, that parental proxy consent to experiments at risks upon their children may validly be given only in cases in which their treatment is in view (as I do, and I understand this is clearer in British medical standards and law than in American) would thus settle for himself the moral verdict concerning much of the research on live human fetuses. There would be no one competent to consent, unless promoting the survival of the fetus was the objective of those investigations. At the least, the presumption would go in that direction, and the burden would be to show why research on fetal human beings should nevertheless be governed by different standards than research on the infant human being. (The entire question of consent and the strange contours of the very notion of authority to consent to fetal research alongside application for an abortion will be explored at length in the final chapter.)

The living previable human fetus may also be likened to an unconscious patient. We shall have to ask, therefore, whether the restrictions upon submitting unconscious patients to research unless it is in their medical interest do not also apply to the fetal human being; and if not, why not?

The previable fetus or still living abortus also closely resembles two other classes of potential human research subjects. In cases of spontaneous abortion of the previable fetus, the fetus resembles the dying. We shall have to ask whether the exclusion of the dying from irrelevant experiments and from research nonbeneficial to them does not apply with equal force to fetal experimentation.

In cases of induced abortion, the fetal human being resembles not only the dying; it also closely resembles the condemned (even if necessarily and justly, but tragically, still the condemned). That, too, should be food for thought as we inquire whether there are some things we ought never to do in order to make medical progress, and to benefit others, and ask ourselves whether fetal research is among those things.

These are some of the themes of research ethics that weave in and out in serious reflection upon the moral issues that have been raised by the availability of this new human research subject in greater numbers today.

Relevant to the morality of this sort of research is also, of course, the question of the morality of abortion. But that ought not be allowed to overshadow the present topic. It is only one theme among others, converging with other themes perhaps, but needing to be sorted out and kept in a subordinate role. On the one hand, we need to note the skewing of a number of the established criteria of research ethics when the climate of abortion is brought into the heart of the matter by some apologists for the morality of fetal research.

On the other hand, those who oppose on moral grounds our current abortion practice will be deeply troubled as they approach the question of the use of the human fetus in experiments useful only to others. Still the thoughtful ones are likely to discern that there is no necessary logical or ethical connection between these two issues. They are apt to analyse their troubled consciences in terms of complicity in a system of which they disapprove, even as sensitive souls in recent years have struggled to separate the good they would do and to which we aspire from involvement in corporate investments in South Africa. For another analogy, LeRoy Walters suggests the following:

> If a particular hospital became the beneficiary of an organized homicide-system which provided a regular supply of fresh cadavers, one would be justified in raising questions about the moral appropriateness of the hospital's continuing cooperation with the suppliers.

Then Walters asks:

> Ought one to make experimental use of the products of an abortion system, when one would object on ethical grounds to many or most of the abortions performed within that system?[2]

That sort of soul searching went on in the Ob-Gyn department of a leading hospital and medical school under religious sponsorship after a quick decision was made to secure a thymus gland, needed to try to save the life of a baby born without immunological competence, from a nearby hospital where thymus glands are readily available because numerous abortions are performed there.

In any case, a simple thought experiment helps to separate these issues. One can imagine that all fetal experimentation is done on still living abortuses obtained from spontaneous abortion or from those abortions he would judge to be justifiable and necessary. Unavoidably the morality of abortion converges with and diverges from other appropriate themes or considerations in any discussion of fetal research. Indeed this ought to be the case.

Still I suggest that someone who believes that it would be wrong to do nontherapeutic research on children, on the unconscious or the dying patient, or on the condemned, may have settled negatively the question of the morality of fetal research, while someone who believes that most abortions performed today are wrong may be tending but he has not yet arrived at an ethical verdict upon that question. An unsound fetal politics falsely proclaims that objections to fetal research stems solely or mainly from moral opposition to the current practice of abortion.

Chapter 4

Research on the Condemned, the Dying, the Unconscious

About 12 or 14 years ago, an American physician, Jack Kevorkian, M.D., published two books and at least one article on a novel use of people who are condemned to die.[1] One book was entitled *Capital Punishment or Capital Gain?* His was a serious proposal in justification of research on the condemned. Even now when capital punishment finds less favor in our society and has been declared unconstitutional under certain circumstances in the United States, it is worth trying to recover the flavor and anatomy of Kevorkian's argument for purposes of comparison with some defenses currently made of experimentation on the live human fetus.

Capital punishment as it existed in 1959–60, Kevorkian believed, offered a "golden opportunity" for research on human beings to break out of the limits imposed by the need to protect normal volunteers from serious damage. He proposed that "a prisoner condemned to death by due process of law be allowed to submit, by his own free choice, to medical experimentation under complete anesthesia (at the time appointed for administering the penalty) as a form of execution in lieu of conventional methods prescribed by law."[2] In fact, the medical experiment, however extreme, need not be thought of as a form of execution, since "ultimate death could be induced by an overdose of anesthetic given by a layman." That is, an official of the state would step in to deliver the *coup de grace.* In case the perilous experiment itself pushed the subject over the brink, Kevorkian contended, physicians would still not be executioners because "their aim was not to kill but to learn."

Likewise it might be argued today that, while some physicians assumed the role of a public functionary (in using socio-economic indices) or the role of executor of women's wishes, still those physicians engaged in fetal research have as such the aim not to kill but to learn. The death decreed by an abortion only affords a "golden opportunity" for "capital gain" for humankind.

The experiments made possible in anticipation of execution, in Kevorkian's judgment, promised "much more than the bleak aim of ending a criminal's life." Likewise, it might be argued today that fetal experiments made possible in anticipation of abortion, or as a consequence of abortive actions set in course, promise much more than the bleak aim of ending the fetus' life. If prenatal lives are going to be wasted anyway, why cannot some of that waste be redeemed?

Moreover, the allocation of funds for much "animal work" now in progress in medical research would be rendered "a complete waste of time and money"; one could proceed at once to the "human work." For Kevorkian the decisive point in favor of his proposal was that rapid progress could be made "in those fields where animal work cannot help (for example, anatomy of the human brain)." That, precisely, is a main apology for the necessity of experimentation on fetuses, namely, that there are uniquely prenatal and pediatric diseases and information about human development in its early stages that finally can only be researched by "human work." Human fetuses already condemned by an abortion decision afford us the same unique opportunity which Kevorkian believed capital punishment opened for human experimentation in general.

In Kevorkian's proposed experiments, it could be argued that "to the condemned" his proposal "allows the dignity inherent in being permitted to decide how he is to die." The condemned are rewarded by a "feeling of utility through death." Some "positive significance" is imparted to the death of his victim if he is a murderer; and Kevorkian believed his proposal afforded "a means of restoring some honor to the family of the condemned." The fact that adults condemned to death are capable of choosing to become heroic partners in medical progress is an advantage condemned fetuses do not have. Here the analogy breaks down.

For society, Kevorkian further argued, the "proposed 'judicial euthanasia' for the first time introduces a concept of recompensing into a matter now of pure vengeance." Likewise, apologists for fetal research sometimes argue that there ought to be some recompense, some good to come from the extraordinary number of unborn lives that today are being destroyed.

A religious interpretation or commentary could not fail to notice at this point the significance of the desire to wrest some recompense or redemption out of the condemnation of these human lives. Surely that motivation has grown enormously among the saving and healing professions and in society generally in face of the huge wastage of one form of human life today by abortion. I believe that a load of guilt is the propellant behind much of the acceptance of fetal research, even as the expected benefits are its lure and goal. If not specific moral guilt, then a load of "survivor guilt"; but surely also a generalized moral guilt as well. The wastage of unborn lives needs redemption; something "must" be saved from it. The research gains promise not only benefits; they also can "rectify" and do at least something to redeem the destruction we collectively are causing in pursuit of other social and personal goods.

Finally, however, Kevorkian guards himself against lending support to capital punishment itself. "The pros and cons of capital punishment are not at all involved in my proposal. My only contention is that so long as it is practiced, and wherever it is practiced, there is a far more humane, sensible and profitable way to administer it." Similar things might be said about the practice of abortion.

Despite its facile persuasiveness, I think we should reject Kevorkian's proposal. Even if his scheme had no tendency to strengthen capital punishment as an institution, it would be morally outrageous for other people to profit by research on the condemned. So also, I suggest, it would be morally outrageous for future fetuses or children to be made to benefit from research on sacrificed fetuses. The research subjects are additionally misused if the experimentation is irrelevant to what caused their condemnation to be deemed just and necessary or electable.

The fetal human being, whether from induced or spontaneous abortion or unsalvageable prematurity, is also among the dying. In research upon the dying we should not, even with their consent, impose on them irrelevant experiments.

With research into cures for their diseases—even beyond any hope of successfully treating their particular case—we reach the outer limit of ethical research upon the dying. This is based on a human being's sense of identity with his body, even with his dying body. Thus Hans Jonas argues[3] that the terminally ill should be spared "the gratuitousness of service to an unrelated cause." In no case should the dying be told: "Since you are here—in the hospital with its facilities—under our care and observation, away from your job (or, perhaps, doomed) we wish to profit from your being available for some other research of great interest we are presently engaged in." Neither ought we to act as if we are saying to the abortus: "Since you are going to die anyway and are available and under observation, wouldn't it be more significant for you to die as our 'partner' in research of great interest and which may prove profitable to the uncondemned?" Research on the terminally ill, Jonas reasoned, should always be relevant to that patient's illness. In research aimed at learning more about that illness, a "residue of identification is left him that it is his own affliction by which he can contribute to the conquest of that affliction." It is a kind of violation of bodily identity, and a misuse of the dying, even to ask the terminally ill to consent to irrelevant research.

A fortiori, we ought not similarly to abuse the fetal research subject who cannot be asked. In the case of the capitally condemned, it generally would not be proposed to limit non-therapeutic research upon them to the development of more humane methods of capital punishment or the accumulation of medical evidence against capital punishment. Nor is fetal research limited to studies intended to remove pain from future abortion procedures or to gather evidence that a civilized society should limit that dying as much as possible. The experiments are irrelevant to the bodily identity or dying of those singled out for coopted contributions to medical progress. They should be spared such gratuitous service. Relevance is the condition that is lacking, and it alone can morally redeem making use of these dying ones.

Doubtless there is an obligation to develop techniques to increase viability and to prevent or offset certain congenital defects or consequences of prematurity. But there can be no obligation—indeed, it would be positively wrong—to obtain those results by means of abortuses who are hovering between life and death precisely because for them no such rescue or remedies were wanted. Those beneficial results should rather be among the research aims of therapeutic investigations that have as a first purpose the promotion of the survival of fetal patients and premature infants.

The fetal subject is also among the unconscious, with the small and, I suggest, morally irrelevant difference that the fetus has never been conscious. Even that concession can be questioned. How accurate it is depends on one's definition of consciousness and at what stage of gestation experiments are proposed to be done on fetuses. The unborn hears the lower tones of its mother's voice and responds to extrauterine stimuli. The fetus is certainly not in coma. There is good evidence that the fetus feels pain, although pain studies are notoriously difficult to do. Perhaps we ought to do pain studies in connection with abortion, if they can be devised, and disseminate that information to the public. If that is possible, the research would be *relevant* to fetal dying, in the sense explained above, even though no one aimed to use the information for the benefit of the particular dying subjects coopted for that purpose.

If the analogy with unconscious patients is believed to be pertinent to an analysis of the moral aspects of fetal research—or to the extent that it is—the conclusion should be clear. To quote Hans Jonas again: "Drafting him [the unconscious] for non-therapeutic experiments is simply and unqualifiedly not permissible; progress or not, he must never be used, on the inflexible principle that utter helplessness demands utter protection."[4] Research on the unconscious subject must be done only in investigations related (however remotely) to his treatment. It is treatment that is the foundation for construing his consent in "Good Samaritan" medicine. If we extend constructive or implied "proxy" consents beyond investigational trials related to treatment, if we also assume that the unconscious subject consents to be used for irrelevant investigations, then we adopt a violent and a false presumption.

Chapter 5

Medical Ethics Skewed
by the Abortion Issue

Earlier I mentioned the fact that a number of the established criteria of research ethics are skewed when abortion is brought into the center of discussions of the morality of fetal research. It is now possible to illustrate this point and give evidence for it, first by reference to a published case study of a fetal research protocol.[1]

The objective in the research was the development of an artificial placenta that would "permit the salvaging of pre-viable or marginally-viable fetuses in the 300 to 1200 gram range." That weight range encompasses many a clearly viable fetus. This must have been a fictional case. Yet there is a wide variability in the gram-weight below which hospitals do not try to salvage newborns. The grave moral issue raised by the lack of approximate agreement in the practice of medicine—entailing that whether a baby will be "given" life depends on the hospital the mother entered—cannot be discussed here.

In the construed case of research, the technique involved cannulating the internal iliac vessels offering total perfusion of the infant. It was anticipated that maintenance of vital signs in the fetal subject would at first be for no more than minutes or hours. Still it was hoped that survival time would increase gradually as the technique was perfected.

So far, so good. But then, we are told, the research team agreed that, until the placenta was a proven lifesaving measure, no fetus would be maintained for more than two weeks because of possible damage to it from the procedure itself. That, I suppose, was a good reason for stopping the experiment. But with that in view, with serious damage to whole living fetuses envisaged, indeed written into the protocol, what were the sufficient justifications for beginning the experiment?

Robert S. Morison of Cornell University, in the discussion of this case, defends the ethics of it. He believes that further threat to the fetus from the procedure is "trivial in comparison" with "a prior finding"—in an abortion decision—"that the right to life of the fetus was outweighed by other considerations." With that, incidentally, Dr. André Hellegers—although he was commenting on fetal research in situ—seemed to agree, when he remarked, "I don't understand why you would want to protect the fetus prior to an abortion. It strikes me as illogical to say you may administer saline, but you may not administer thalidomide or drug X690" to test its damage to the fetus.[2]

Is it possible, however, to separate the morality of abortion from the morality of fetal research? Can we prescind from Morison's approval of abortion and Hellegers' opposition to it? This might be done in the present case, as I suggested above, by supposing that the research was to be done only on spontaneously aborted fetuses and on justifiably aborted fetuses—those abortions Hellegers or anyone else would say were just and necessary.

But then, on this supposition, the distinction between nontherapeutic and remotely possible therapeutic investigations on live abortuses returns with a vengeance to control all sound ethical reasoning on this subject. The cruciality of this distinction is disclosed by the contradiction—the dilemma—that lies at the heart of attempts to justify nonbeneficial research on still living abortuses. One must agree with the odd conclusion of Dr. Morison that "a new and serious problem" will arise as and to the degree that experiments on the aborted for the sake of other unborns or infants "approach success":

It would clearly be unethical to employ extraordinary means actually to bring into the world of the living an infant whose parents had already rejected it. In other words, as soon as the experiments give promise of imminent success, they should be limited to those spontaneously aborted fetuses that the parents wish to bring to maturity.

That says in so many words that the more certain we are that benefits will accrue *only* to society or to other fetuses and the more the still-living abortus alone will be damaged or suffer pain or injury, the more we should approve the research; that the closer socially beneficial experimentation comes to bestowing some benefit also on the research subject, the more it deserves moral condemnation. That reverses the ordinary canons of medical ethics.

Morison seems to believe that a fetus has no claims on medical practice if its parents have already rejected it. A prior abortion decision has replaced the ordinary canons of research ethics. Parents' wishes make abortion moral; they also determine that *the research* is moral, provided the experimenters stay within the range of the woman's sovereign decision. Dr. Kurt Hirschhorn said that if it is not possible to make this fetus into a child, we therefore can consider it as nothing more than a piece of tissue. I think it fair to observe that Dr. Morison says, in effect, that since we cannot make this fetus into a wanted child, we therefore can consider it as nothing more than a piece of tissue. The experiment in question might make this fetus into a child. The protocol forfended that "danger" because of damage to that possible child. Dr. Morison wants primarily to avoid making an unwanted fetal human being into an unwanted child. So for him it would be morally outrageous for one of these experiments to succeed or to approach success—threatening "to bring into the world of the living an infant" whose value has not been derived from someone's evaluation of or interest in it. By contrast, as we shall see, the original NIH policy proposal affirms that "the decision of the Supreme Court on abortion does not eliminate the ethical issues involved in research on the nonviable human fetus."

What, then, is left in the foregoing case if we strip from it the permissiveness illicitly supposed to flow from someone's elective abortion decision or from the legalities? Suppose the experiments were to be done only on whole still-living fetuses resulting from spontaneous abortions (or from "just and necessary" abortions). The abortuses would, then, be condemned by no human intervention (or by an entirely justifiable one); yet they would still be entitatively alive in important and relevant ways, or else the research would be pointless. What then?

I suggest that the paradox at the heart of abortus research would still remain. This would be unconsented, irrelevant research on the dying (unless for the purpose of saving them). It would still be research on the, tragically, "condemned." It would be seizing the "golden opportunity" helplessly afforded by those about to die for the sake of those who may yet live. We would be thrown back upon the clear provisions of the protocol in this case, which warned of the danger that possibly seriously injurious "nonbeneficial" research might become "successful" too soon. Without waiting for any parents' wishes to bring fetuses to maturity and without excuse from anybody's rejection of them, the provision must be (if the dying are to be *used* for the living) that, at least "during the critical period of transfer of the fetus to the artificial placenta, no fetus . . . be maintained for more than a two-week period because of possible damage" to the human research subject from the procedure itself. Disposal must be arranged in advance. As Sumner B. Twiss, Jr., wrote in the discussion of this case, it would "appear that the researchers are trying to rectify one moral wrong by performing another."

I see no way to remove the ethical contradiction from the heart of that research on whole, still living fetuses: the closer such experiments come to being lifesaving or beneficial to the subject, the clearer it becomes that the use of still-living fetuses who could not possibly benefit and who might even be harmed by the trial was wrong in the first place. Only possibly beneficial experiments on the still living can without an understanding consent be justified, or at least no experiments whose risks of injury are not negligible and/or those whose objective is to promote the survival of the subject. The proposal is to do damaging or highly risky experiments upon the dying, i.e. the still-living nonviable fetus, precisely in order to make rapid medical progress. *Incidentally,* abortion makes these dying available. No one's views on the morality of abortion alters or can remove the offensiveness of such research practiced on the dying. The prohibition would hold even if all abortions were morally justified.

The ordinary canons of medical ethics are also put in disarray by ascribing cruciality to abortion in prospect. This can be seen from an examination of an article by Dr. Willard Gaylin and Dr. Marc Lappé, entitled "Fetal Politics."[3] The framestory of that article is a two-part moral argument. The first element is legal positivism. The second element is a very odd line of reasoning I can only call the "slip-back-up-the-moral-slope" argument, or a "one-wrong-justifies-a-lesser-wrong" argument.

By legal positivism I mean, of course, the Supreme Court's abortion decision. That is a *fact*. The widespread practice of medically unnecessary abortion is also a *fact,* made legal by the factual sway of that legal decision. From no legal "is" can a moral "ought" be drawn—either in medical or in general ethics. The superiority of the original NIH guidelines, we shall see, is most clearly evident because the drafters proceeded to reason *ethically* about fetal research and the needed guidelines, the Supreme Court notwithstanding. The inferiority of its subsequent revision is clear from its crucial introduction of legal positivism and the facticity of abortion. To say this is *not* to say the Court's decision was morally wrong. It is only to say that from the fact of it—or even from the *legal* rightness of it—no conclusion follows for morality or for the ethical practice of medicine.

Gaylin and Lappé do not so conclude. Legal positivism works to produce a line of moral reasoning only in combination with the second ingredient in their argument. They write:

> Affording the fetus the same protection as the child (both innocent and non-consenting subjects) seems ludicrous in the light of prevailing public acceptance and government approval of abortion. In abortion we more or less readily condone procedures which subject the fetus to dismemberment, salt-induced osmotic shock, or surgical extirpation; certainly no conceivable experiment would do the same. Yet wholesale acceptance of the procedures of abortion and rejection of those of experimentation is precisely the current moral stance of the federal government. Mere consistency would seem to demand that society cannot condone

abortion procedures which must subject the live fetus to unimaginable acts of violence, and then balk at giving a mother an aspirin prior to those procedures in order to determine if the drug crosses placenta—with hopes, thereby, that the knowledge will prevent damage to future wanted babies.

Now, why is that passage persuasive while at the same time in sound moral logic it is unconvincing? Everything depends on whether the second element in this two-part argument has any reasonable weight as an ethical argument. These writers' justification of the morality of fetal research (given the positive legality of abortion) entirely depends not on "mere consistency" but on whether it is correct in ethical reasoning to argue that one wrong justifies another (in the special form that one wrong justifies a lesser one).

In oral discussion of this issue, one of these authors (Gaylin) put the point as follows (stressing that he was choosing his words carefully): Since *we have given ourselves the right* to medically unnecessary abortion [given ourselves the right to do to the fetus those "unimaginable acts of violence" to which the above passage vividly refers], then *we have given ourselves the right* to place the fetus at risk of lesser injury. That is why we "cannot" now "balk."

The aspirin begs the question, since one might justify such research because comparatively benign on wanted unborns or with children. In any case, that example goes in the direction of justifying fetal research by means of refined distinctions concerning the benignity of the procedure, not by crucial reference to the abortion in prospect. A justification of fetal research requires concentration elsewhere than on abortion in prospect or than on the mere legality of abortion.

Gaylin did not say: Since current abortion-practice is *right,* so also is potentially harmful fetal research in anticipation of abortion. He did not say only that since abortion is *legal* in positive law, so also fetal research should be legal; nor at this point did he expressly appeal to legal positivism alone, to say that both could be right because legal. Instead he appealed to realities behind the law which the present law on abortion covers. We have by law given ourselves the right to do these background unimaginable acts of violence in abortion procedures; we then can legitimately claim the right to do lesser possible harm for the sake of other wanted babies. If that contention has any force at all, the argument more than borders on saying: Since we have given ourselves the right to do wrong, we have given ourselves the right to do other, lesser wrongs. That has to be the force of language carefully chosen to set aside those more superficial appeals to the mere facticity of abortion practice or solely to legal positivism. This is what skews the ordinary canon of medical ethics: do no harm.

But the foregoing puts moral reasoning into disarray. One harm cannot justify another, nor two wrongs make a right—even if the second harm or wrong is less than the first. Here we have the oddity of a "slip-back-up-the-moral-slope" argument. The mere consistency invoked is actually to use one sort of harmfulness to move on to another that is now procedurally permitted or opened by the first.

That ingredient in the two-part "argument" won't work. And since the appeal to legal positivism won't work either as a moral argument, the passage and article in which these appeals are intertwined—each needing the failed support of the other—won't work as moral argument. It amounts to an exercise in persuasion. Two bad arguments do not make a correct one.

Here a religious commentary brings to light the pervasive sense of collective guilt concerning our current abortion practice. This helps us to understand one important element in the persuasiveness of this sort of argumentation. Collectively guilt-laden, we go on (like the Dostoevsky's character Stavrogin in *The Possessed*) to other potential harms and wrongs in order to avoid acknowledging the first (with the small but significant difference that Stavrogin was impelled to go on to more heinous wrongs, he determined his personality to plunge down the moral slope, while we propose to move back up it). We are determined to wrest by our scientific works some good out of guilt-laden harmfulness to unborn life.

In their discussion of "the good case" to be made for fetal

research, Gaylin and Lappé use the salvic language we should learn to expect in these matters. Experimentation, they write, can "ennoble" the death of the doomed fetus if it is utilized "to serve its more fortunate fellows." That "ennoblement," they say, brings fetal research "closest to the therapeutic model." Gaylin and Lappé write that "at worst fetal research degrades abortion by making it a vehicle for ends of no relevance to the specific life it takes; at best, however, it endows the process of abortion with human values it will not otherwise have." That is what they mean in condoning fetal research that is "close to the therapeutic model," i.e. in the service of fellow fetuses. I say that is close to a "salvation model." But then for us moderns therapy *is* salvation.

More important to say in rejoinder, the doomed fetus is in need of no substitute therapy, no substitute human values, no need of salvation, ennoblement, or redemption. It is rather we who do not save it from needless doom, and we alone, who are searching for some therapy for our collective souls, some ennoblement, some source of solace from, nonspecific, guilt. It is "the process of abortion" and the individual and collective agents of it, who desperately need to be endowed with human values we and abortion will not otherwise have.

I do not mean to impute my memory of Gaylin's oral statement of his position to Gaylin and Lappé as joint authors. We need therefore to return to the article on "Fetal Politics" to find, if possible, verification of the foregoing analysis. Place side by side with the appeal in the passage quoted on pp. 41–42, the following passage that makes the same point or appeal:

There is an element of the irrational about [current efforts to ban fetal research] that perplexes many of us. Does it not seem hypocritical for a country like the United States which has neglected the nutritional and hygenic requisites for healthy wanted pregnancies to the point that it ranks fourteenth in infant mortality to be so concerned about potential damage to never-to-be-born fetuses. How is it that a Congress that moves so slowly in major areas of health concern, that has turned its back for the fourth time in a row on its simple obligation to protect the public from the poisons introduced into its environment and food by over-zealous commercial interests, has had the temerity to leap into this nettle of unresolved dilemmas?

Into the nettle it jumped, given the vacuum in medical ethics and regulation. Surely, however, as a *formal* matter, Congress can be right one time and not in many other of its actions and inactions—whether it was or was not wrong or precipitous in this instance. Many wrongs do not make right right or wrong wrong, even as two harms do not add up to an ethical justification. I have heretofore found such persuasive appeals more common among religious than among scientific authors.

The important thing, however, is to ask whether the appeals —let us no longer call them moral arguments—made by these two passages are not identical. Because child neglect is so wrong, it is ludicrous to "balk" at fetal research: that is the "argument." In the one case, it is the terrible harmfulness of nutritional and other neglects and inaction that seems glaringly inconsistent with concern to protect the fetal human research subject. In the other case, it is the unimaginable acts of extirpation of the fetus that make that concern seem ludicrous to these authors.

That is all well and good if the point was to use persuasive rhetoric to get leverage to "change the system" or to correct the woeful harms cited. Such, however, was not the point of the argument. The point was rather to argue from the ghastly damage to infants allowed and the extirpation done to fetuses in our society to a moral justification of potentially harmful fetal research. The formal ethical argument is in each case the same; and it is fatally flawed.

I am inclined to agree with these authors that an unskewed medical ethics would lead rather to the requirement that choice of the method of abortion be not made by simply balancing considerations that affect morbidity to the mother alone. That should also include a requirement that the fetus not be subjected to prolonged and unduly stressful injury, as is now the case with salt-poisoning induced by saline abortions. Perhaps it is too much to expect today that there be awakened in public and in medical conscience a strong concern over the comparative humaneness of abortion procedures. To say the least, however, an unskewed medical ethics does not lead in the direction of *adding* deliberately induced harmfulness to the fetus—on the excuse that it is "part" of the abortion procedure (as in DHEW-NIH revised guidelines, to be examined in detail in Chapter 9 below).

Gaylin and Lappé's framework moral argument—and it is intended to be such—is repeated at the end of the article. Since we know anyway that we are going to destroy, dismember, and discard the fetus in a procedure known as abortion it seems a "small indignity" to expose it to rubella vaccine just prior of that termination. Here again, one indignity justifies another, provided only that the former is the larger one. In the experiment in question, physicians needed to know whether rubella vaccine will harm the fetus if unknowingly pregnant women are vaccinated. There was no other "safe" way to get that information except by trying it on women in anticipation of abortion. But of course, if the ordinary canons of medical ethics had not already been skewed by ascribing cruciality to abortion in prospect, and if "do no harm" controlled the manner in which the vaccine was brought into use, a way could have been found to do no harm either way. Surely, in the period of the vaccine's introduction to the adult population of women, that concern and medicine's concern to do no harm would indicate a brief period of refraining from sexual intercourse to avoid vaccination while pregnant. As Gaylin and Lappé point out in their discussion of this case, we now largely avoid the dilemma by vaccinating preadolescent girls or the population of gradeschoolers instead of women of childbearing age exposed to danger of pregnancy (if that is a proper manner of speaking). So we did not need to "ennoble" the death of doomed fetuses. There were alternative ways of saving other more fortunate fetuses without obtaining that information by possibly harming and using the condemned.

A final case-oriented statement of the argument we are examining has to do with the destruction of a normal male fetus (whose sex only can be determined by amniocentesis) 50 percent of the time rather than the male fetus afflicted with hemophilia in order to prevent one child suffering from that disease. Gaylin and Lappé write:

> We find ourselves therefore in this peculiar position. The destruction of one or two normal fetuses to protect against one abnormal fetus under current law in the United States is not legally objectionable. We allow and sometimes encourage such a practice in the case of a male fetus at risk for hemophilia. Here, an abortion of the normal male (usually undistinguishable from its affected brother) is sanctioned to ensure that half the time a hemophilic male is eliminated. Yet to do research on a *fetus that is about to be destroyed* which might save both infants, if we accept the current status quo, is morally objectionable.

Now, I submit that the appeal to the destruction of a normal male fetus, in order to ensure that half the time an afflicted hemophilic male is prevented from being born to a life of suffering, gathers strength because it appeals to our *sense of injustice*. To do that is rather like operating on the wrong patient, and defending that tragic mistake by saying that for the right patient the operation would have been a success. These authors need to accept the current moral status quo and hold that unalterable, with the sense of injustice it awakens, in order to use it as a launching pad to the conclusion that at worst fetal research is a lesser evil.

They summarize: "The medical ethics 'do no harm' would, of course, be violated [by fetal research]—but we have already violated that principle when we accept the concept of abortion. The ultimate harm of destroying the fetus trivializes that which precedes it." Perhaps, indeed, it is true that current abortion practice is in grave violation of that cardinal medical ethical principle. That is not the issue here. In considering the morality of fetal research, however, it is precisely the wrongfulness and harmfulness of abortion that has to be held as a premise in this attempt to reach a justification of the lesser harm or wrong that may be entailed in experimentation on fetuses when abortion is in prospect. The contention has no force unless abortion truly is an "unimaginable act of violence" (as, for example, tissue research is not). In turn, my reply has been that, even so, the ethical "argument" won't work because an established harm possesses no tendency to justify later harm, two wrongs do not make a right, a greater wrong does not help to justify a lesser one. This is a formal matter that remains true in the logic of moral discourse whether abortion is right or wrong, and whether fetal research can otherwise be justified or not. There may be valid arguments for the morality of experimentation on fetuses, but this one is not.

When Gaylin and Lappé introduce their "good case" of a sort of fetal research they believe to be most readily warrantable, they set out to establish a minimum case. They want to allow that some fetal research is unnecessary and perhaps immoral. They do not even undertake to describe the entire range of research that seems likely to be morally acceptable to a reasonable majority of people.

On closer scrutiny, however, the claim that theirs is a minimalist case is exceedingly weak if not entirely nugatory. For the governing stipulation is that fetal research be devoted to progress in the future medical care of the doomed fetus' more fortunate siblings. Indeed, the point at which it becomes unethical not to do fetal experimentation is reached "when the research has as its objective the saving of the lives (or the reduction of defects) of *other* wanted fetuses."

Now, is that limitation minimalist or maximalist? It seems minimalist, in that fetuses are not to be coopted for the conquest of mankind's general ills but only for those afflicting other prenatal or newborn lives. Yet in terms of the "argument" we have reviewed, within that extrinsic limitation there is a qualitatively "maximalist case" that would be justified. If abortion in prospect is deemed to be crucial in the moral argument for fetal research, then such experimentation need entail no "small indignity" to the doomed fetus, but only one *smaller* than "extirpation" and "unimaginable acts of violence." So in principle and in the logic of the moral argument, *anything* done that might yield knowledge fruitful for other wanted fetuses here finds justification in principle and not only small indignities, some risks, unexpected injury, etc. To push the maximalism entailed in their line of reasoning, I know, would be to ignore the moral sensibilities of both these authors. But then I simply must say that they are better men than their arguments.

The fact is that we have here a replication of the standard "solution" routinely proposed by contemporary American researchers. Experimentation with children (having no bearing on their treatment) is said to be justified if limited to research on uniquely pediatric diseases; and now experimentation with the fetus is deemed not only necessary but right if limited to the study of uniquely fetal or neonatal diseases. That limitation, which is almost automatically forthcoming from the medical profession, is, I am inclined to think, a fig leaf that covers the unseemly parts of a compromise ethics—a compromise between benefits-to-come and "doing no harm."

I may be wrong in that judgment. Significant to note, however, is that such a limitation upon morally permissible research is for other reasons held minimalist in the case of research using children, because the child might be injured and still live; while in the case of fetuses the very same limitation knows no bounds if abortion in prospect is taken to be crucial. The upshot of that would be to say *in principle* that no indignity, no injury, no harm that may be believed useful to other less fortunate fetuses need be morally prohibited. That puts us back at Kevorkian's proposal for research on the capitally condemned. They may be pushed to the brink of anything short of experimental execution. And that I judge to be "irrational," "ridiculous," "ludicrous," or, better said, morally outrageous.

No one seriously says this, of course; not Gaylin and Lappé. Nor anyone when pasting the justificatory label "for the sake of other fetuses" or "for the sake of other children" on experimentation on innocent, nonconsenting, or indeed condemned or dying fetal human subjects.

Then the covering of the only seemingly important justificatory category "for the sake of other fetuses or newborns" ought to be abandoned—or at least reduced to a quite subordinate role. For one thing, I see no sound or compelling reason to deny the doomed fetus the privilege of having its death "ennobled" by contributing to the betterment of humankind generally and the conquest of all our diseases—if, for example, no fetal research is under way in the medical center, they would otherwise be wasted in the incinerator, or if general medical progress could be very rapidly advanced by experimentation on fetuses in anticipation of abortion without that restriction. It is, indeed, a compromise arrangement. One could ask what is the purpose of it in the moral history of mankind: for the protection of the human subject or as balm for our consciences? If benefits alone justify, they justify a research practice without that limitation. Since we nevertheless cherish this compromise, we may secretly know that benefits alone justify very little in the moral life.

More important, that routine justification hides from view more significant limitations that are actually operative in medical research on unconsenting subjects: the degrees of possible harm or risks; how discernible they should be, and so on. These judgments need to be debated, carefully refined, and formulated for research practice, if that is a moral rule-governed activity protective of human subjects. Such careful analysis is necessary if some forms of fetal research should ever be deemed ethical. Everyone's attention is taken from that issue and task when abortion is alleged to be in any way related to possible right-making features of fetal research. If that error does not tempt us to maximalist permissions, it still blunts discriminations where discriminations are due, and which need to be shown to be ethically decisive—if all fetal research should not be judged to be simply wrong.

The superiority of the original NIH effort at medical ethical rule-making is evident in the fact that it proceeded to give primacy to the principle, Do no harm—the Supreme Court notwithstanding. That point of view leads to morally significant distinctions between experiments to determine harm to the fetus and the testing of benign or helpful substances at the placental passage. It leads to questions about discernible risks, discernibly no risks, etc., and to debate about them. The inferiority of the subsequent revision is evident in that it dismissed the criteria of additional risk or harm when abortion is or is nearly coincident. To that a proper reply is, two coincident harms—the one to the unborn, the other to the fetal research subject, where they are the same life—cannot make a right.

Chapter 6

Fetal Research in Utero:
The NIH Provisional Guidelines

The Peel Report (1972) was not content simply with using stipulations on the safe side of viability to define a new class of human research subjects, as in the main were the American reports and deliberations in progress at about that same time (1971–72). Wishing, obviously, to legitimate some sorts of fetal studies, it nevertheless circumscribed them with far more than procedural rules. With regard to research on the fetus in situ, for example, the Peel Report states quite categorically, "it is unethical to administer drugs or carry out any procedures during pregnancy with the deliberate intent of ascertaining the harm that these might do to the fetus." To much the same effect, the NIH guidelines (November 1973) requires that "no experimental procedures entailing risk to the fetus be undertaken in anticipation of abortion."

Is there any difference in the force or meaning of those two prohibitions? "With the deliberate intent of ascertaining the harm that these might do to the fetus" could be regarded as less restrictive than "entailing risk to the fetus." Still in a criminal or civil suit, a British researcher under one guideline and an American researcher under the other would likely be held to approximately the same standards, because in the first case the physician would be held accountable for what he expertly knew might harm (so what was the purpose of his research if not to ascertain that?) while in the second case the physician could be shown, on expert testimony, to know that most medical interventions entail some risks.

More significant is the fact that in both policies something is categorically forbidden to be done for the sake of beneficial consequences to come for other unborns, infants or children. So much so, that the NIH guideline (in language the more restrictive of the two) declares that experimentation entailing risk to the fetus in situ in anticipation of abortion is a "null class" among possible ways to advance medical knowledge. While ordinarily physicians insist that any medical intervention entails some risks, physician-researchers, naturally enough, commonly say that their experiments involving young or otherwise incompetent human subjects involve no risks, or no substantial risks. Taking all these matters into account, I judge that the British and the American guidelines forbid the administration or testing of drugs like thalidomide that palpably may harm. However, on some constructions, the NIH guidelines might permit the scientific testing of whether certain beneficial substances cross the placental barrier from one blood stream to another with no or little risk of harm to the fetus.

The NIH guideline forbidding risky research on the fetus in utero in anticipation of abortion is supported by two considerations. One is "the right of every woman to change her decision regarding abortion." The Peel Report in no way refers to the woman's change of mind. It does mention the researcher's risk of prosecution if the fetus is delivered alive and harmed. The Peel provision forbidding procedures having the deliberate intent of ascertaining the harm that those might do to the fetus brushes aside both the fact of anticipated abortion and the woman's consent (a fortiori her change of mind is excluded from consideration). The provision continues: "notwithstanding that arrangements may have been made to terminate the pregnancy and even if the mother is willing to consent to such an experiment." The foundation for medicine's duty to "do no harm" to the fetus rests rather on the Peel Report's interpretation of the criminal law in the preceding paragraph: "the protection afforded to the fetus is continuous and is not abrogated by the fact that it may be the intention at the time of the affliction of the injury that the fetus should be prevented by a subsequent abortion from attaining life." Thus, medicine's obligation to do no harm remains in full effect, and nothing depends on either planned abortion or on anyone's consent or will.

Besides taking into account the woman's possible change of mind, the American guideline is based also on another justifying reason, and notably this comes first in the sequence of reasons given. "The recent decision of the Supreme Court on abortion does not nullify," so far as medicine is concerned, "the ethical obligation to protect the developing fetus from avoidable harm." This obligation, "along with" the woman's right to change her decision regarding abortion, leads to a strict proscription of research that may injure the fetus. The latter cannot be justified by the excuse that the abortion planned is a still more serious injury, or by reasoning that an abortion, since it eliminates the damagee, will of course eliminate any damage that might have resulted from the fetal experimentation itself.

The preamble paragraph of this section of the NIH notice of proposed policies for the protection of human subjects states the first "good reason" for forbidding fetal research in anticipation of abortion in the strongest possible terms and without qualification. To put the two reasons together in proper sequence, the NIH guideline states that the medical obligation "to protect the developing fetus from avoidable harm . . . *along with* the right of every woman to change her decision regarding abortion" (italics added) forbid fetal experiments in utero in anticipation of abortion. The words "along with" may, indeed, weaken the prohibition if that means that these considerations are good reasons only when taken together, or that if the woman had no right or is unlikely to change her mind, the physician's obligation to protect the fetus from avoidable harm would disappear.

On its face, however, the appeal to the protection of life whatever its age or circumstances is the stronger and more universal appeal. That depends on no one's arbitrary liberty. Moreover, the policy does not state that the "child-to-be" should be protected from avoidable harm—which would be the appropriate language if the woman's possible change of mind was the operative test. It says protect the "fetus," not a possible future infant, from avoidable harm. Furthermore, the preamble paragraph lays down the following general principle of medical ethics: "Respect for the dignity of human life must not be compromised whatever the age, circumstance, or *expectation of life of the individual*. Therefore, all appropriate procedures providing protection for children as subjects in biomedical research must be applied with equal rigor and with additional safeguards to the fetus" (italics added).

The operative clause in that initial statement of the moral standard to be used in appraising fetal research is the verdict that respect for human life should not vary with the "expectation of life of the individual." That applies with "equal rigor" to the fetus. Thus medical ethical approval cannot be given to potentially harmful experimentation upon the condemned, because they are condemned, or upon the dying, because they have not long to live. So "with equal rigor and with additional safeguards to the fetus," there can be no potentially harmful fetal research "in anticipation of abortion." Respect for the dignity of human life must not be compromised simply because the fetus has not long to live. A task of medicine is to protect the developing fetus, even so, from "avoidable harm."

Thus in regard to this first kind of fetal experiment, we have here an admirable application of the ethics of medical care to a new sort of circumstance that, if those principles could be bent or broken, promises more rapid advancement of knowledge and benefit to others. Whether or not one agrees with this judgment, the considerations applied in this case and the weights assigned each should be clear.

However, let us now make an hypothesis contrary to the plain language of the NIH guidelines. Let us suppose a "softer" reading by positing that only the woman's right or likelihood of changing her mind about a planned abortion forbids the physician-researcher from submitting the fetus, with her consent, to medical experimentation, since if she changes her mind and the fetus is subsequently born it may have suffered avoidable harm for which the researcher can be held responsible.

If this were the meaning of the NIH guideline, only the possibility of a last-minute reprieve tells against potentially harmful (and potentially profitable) experimentation on the condemned fetus. This softer reading would contradict what we said above: it would hold that "fetus" was not really meant, but rather "child-to-be" or "future possible infant." In the however unlikely event that the woman changes her mind, the future child should have been protected from even remotely possible harm. So, contrary to the plain language used, "expectation of life," however small, is precisely the qualifier to be taken into account in the case of a condemned, but not yet executed, fetus in situ. That "expectation of life" remains in force as a consideration in the case of planned abortion because, but only because, in the event the woman changes her mind she may yet grant the condemned fetus expectations that are not now in view; and, if she does this, the child may be irrevocably damaged.

Now, I cannot prove that the woman's right to a possible change of mind was not the crux of the matter for the drafters of the NIH document. If it was, however, they were poor drafters. The sequence of the reasons they offered and the words "along with," which seemed to subordinate a woman's changeability about abortion to the better of two reasons for forbidding fetal experiments begun in situ—together with the forceful expressions used that go to support a stronger reading —were meant simply to show that the drafters had touched all the ethical bases. The claim of the fetus to protection from avoidable harm was invoked only in passing. On this interpretation, the woman's right to a possible change of mind has, first, to be given its proper weight; only thereafter do we need to give any consideration to the protection of the fetus in medical ethics. If such was actually the meaning of the drafters, then suspicion of conscious or unconscious "bad faith" must surround everything said in the policy statement about respect for human life regardless of its age, circumstance, or the individual's "expectation of life," applied "with equal rigor and with additional safeguards" to the fetus.

On the "softer" reading, which seems strained and implausible to me, the following would be the consequence in specific cases of fetal research begun in situ. On this view, a woman's possible change of mind is the thing that alone makes operative any consideration of protecting the fetus from avoidable harm, and her changeability is the sole reason for not taking the fetus' present short life-expectancy into account in planning to experiment on him.

But then the woman's *likelihood* of changing her mind would seem to be, within limits, a researchable matter. That would be a slender reed on which to hang the categorical prohibition of fetal research in situ in anticipation of abortion announced by this proposed policy. Such a conclusion would seem to vary as its sole condition varies, or might be determined empirically to vary. A sliding scale would surely be used: as the woman becomes more settled in her choice of abortion, her fetus would become more eligible for possibly harmful experimentation in situ.

To be noted, especially, is the fact that as the moment of the scheduled abortion approaches, the more permissible fetal research in situ in anticipation of abortion would become. It might even be said that, according to this "softer" reading, the NIH guideline has either not addressed itself to the question of fetal experimentation begun at about the time of abortion and concluded during or shortly after the abortion, or else that it means silently to approve of it [Type (2) above]. That, in turn, would entail that the NIH guideline meant to endorse potentially harmful or painful fetal experimentation precisely when the "expectation of life" of the research subject becomes *assuredly* short. The more condemned the subject, the freer the research would be from any limits. That paradoxically is the very opposite of the meaning usually understood by the medical ethical principle that "respect for the dignity of human life must not be compromised whatever the . . . expectation of life of the individual," which this report affirms at the outset should be applied rigorously to the fetus.

But let us pursue this reading no longer. We should turn rather to the moral weight that ought or ought not be assigned to a woman's "right" to change her mind in such a case. It seems clear that a woman, once having knowingly consented to potentially harmful research on her fetus in situ in anticipation of abortion, thereby restricted her future liberty; she impaired her subsequent right to change her mind about the planned abortion even if she might not have waived that right altogether. For the whole alleged point of some sorts of fetal research is the need for condemned fetuses who can be submitted to graver risks of more serious induced injuries than we would inflict, for example, on infants. If a woman consented to that and the injurious experiment had been begun, who among us would say she still has an unimpaired right to change her mind? Even if she had an arbitrary liberty to abort, we would not say she has an arbitrary liberty to injure and then to change her mind about abortion. To say that she still would have an arbitrary liberty in exercise would be to say she has a right knowingly to do injury to a child she is bringing into the world, and that she remains master of that total line of actions from beginning to end.

We shall return to the intriguing general question, Who consents to fetal research in an abortion situation? in the final chapter.

Chapter 7

Live Abortus Research:
The NIH Provisional Guidelines

To its credit, the Peel Report did not stop after its beginning of a definition of the human fetal research subject by the stipulation of measurements on the safe side of viability. It went on to issue some sound principles governing research on such human subjects. The NIH guidelines do that also, but without explicitly stating any measurable parameters for this new class of subjects. That may be an unfinished conceptual task: the definition of a new sort of human research subject that is live enough not to be dead, not yet mature enough to be an infant, yet a human being enough to deserve protections. The sound practical guidelines in both documents presume that we possess such a definition.

Even in such an unfinished definition, the line between pre-viability and viability seems clear enough. It is expressly stated for research purposes in the Peel Report and left to the discretion of physicians in the NIH guidelines. Thus the Peel Report declares that "when the fetus is viable after delivery, the ethical obligation is to sustain its life so far as possible, and it is both immoral and illegal to carry out any experiments on it which are inconsistent with treatment necessary to promote its life." The NIH policy reads: "If there is a reasonable possibility that the life of the fetus may be saved, experimental and established methods may be used to achieve that goal."

Initially I was troubled by the use of that expression "may be used," entailing, it seemed to me, too much discretionary latitude left to physicians. The Peel version is more forceful: it states that if a viable fetus is delivered—presumably even after an abortion—the physician's overriding responsibility is from that point no longer to the mother alone but also to promote the neonate's life. The American guidelines state that if an aborted fetus is possibly viable, life-supporting techniques *may* be employed. That does seem a weaker expression of a physician's duty.

Nevertheless, LeRoy Walters[1] has persuaded me that both guidelines mean to establish a single, universalizable standard for the treatment of all viable or possibly viable prematures (whether from abortion or not). He formulates that standard in the following general rule: "Treat all viable or potentially viable fetuses equally, regardless of the circumstances of their delivery." The "may" in the American guidelines is not there to permit discriminations in violation of the foregoing principle. It rather recognizes the discretion any physician must exercise in judging whether lifesaving techniques are truly "indicated," or are useless, or would only severely retard the premature. He must do this regardless of the circumstances that delivered the fetus into his hands. If the Peel Report seems more stringent, we ought to remember that it is perfectly possible for a physician to walk away and wait for only a few minutes until the gram weight of a living abortus drops from 301 to 299. It then becomes an eligible subject in research that is inconsistent with (or at least that fails to offer) treatment to promote life. We who once were fellow fetuses were once also helpless in the hands of an ethical or an unethical physician. It is impossible and may be undesirable to remove his discretion.

But if the "research imperative" is not to lead physicians into the temptation to treat potentially viable abortuses dissimilarly from other living fetuses and, what is more important, if physician-researchers mean not only to do right but also to be seen to do so, then they should be the first to call for the instatement in American fetal research policy of something like the stringent definition of "viability" in the British guidelines.

For, in the above instance, a physician's "discretion" to walk away until gram weight falls and he has an eligible research subject can in principle be exercised only within the stringent measurable limits of "20 weeks, 300 grams." He is told when to research and when not to research, even if he is not told all he needs to decide about when lifesaving efforts are to be used for fetuses in general. Perhaps, as Walters argued, the American guidelines *mean* to say: Treat viable and potentially viable fetuses equally, regardless of the circumstances of their delivery. Still the objective meaning of "previable" for research purposes needs to be made clear, if physicians are to be protected from having too much liberty to mix research goals with their proper discretion in promoting the life of immatures.

In the background here is a potential and staggering conflict between maternal intention to abort and an ethical physician's duty to save human life. The guidelines, however, did not create that collision; in providing rules governing fetal research they are formulating the terms of that collision. In fact they help to inform the conscience and guide the discretion of physicians so that such a collision becomes morally unavoidable for them. The task of trying to harmonize medical care for young life with the "research imperative" ethically is, at one and the same time, a task of trying to bring that same ethical research into harmony with the practice of abortion. An abortus that can be saved is excluded from the class of research subjects. There may still be a potential collision at the line of viability even when the research meaning of that line is drawn so as to put the physician on notice always to promote survival whenever he can, because a judgment that this is the case in a particular instance must still be discretionary (i.e. prudent). Still an attempted abortion does not weaken a physician's obligation to respect and protect life. He should treat similarly all fetuses that similarly evidence potential viability.

With respect to abortus research (live, intact abortuses that are previable), the NIH guidelines fill in, implicitly at least, the parameters of the definition of this new class of human research subject by their reference to "signs of life" earlier than viability. In introducing our topic, the American guidelines specifically exclude from the meaning of "live" abortus research "the placenta, fetal material which is mascerated at the time of expulsion, a dead fetus [sic], and isolated fetal tissue or organs excised from a dead fetus." Thus, on the one side we have a line drawn between a previable and a viable fetus or abortus; on the other side, a plain distinction made between a certainly previable abortus and a dead one. Use of the latter in research falls, along with mascerated tissue and the use of isolated organs, under other standards. So here we have an entity too alive to be dead, not mature enough to be a viable baby, yet human enough to be specially protectable.

I said earlier that there might be an unfinished conceptual task for our rational reflection in the matter of fetus/abortus research. The conceptual task may be near completion, in the light of those "signs of life" which the NIH guidelines go on to say ought to be respected and never violated in the not-dead, previable abortus. Taking these into account, the remaining task for us is to resist the enormous pressures to define eligibility for ethically unlimited research procedures simply in terms of fetal salvageability.

Within this outline of a class of human beings, the NIH guidelines prohibit certain actions from ever being done to the intact living abortus—not for any possible research benefits to come. That policy declares in general terms that while research must go forward, the research imperatives must first be in conformity with "ethical standards": "Such research," it states, "must meet ethical standards as well as show a clear relation either to the expectation of saving the life of premature infants through the development of rescue techniques, or to the furthering of our knowledge of human development and thereby our capacity to offset the disabilities associated with prematurity."

It is the attending physician, not the investigator, who must determine the viability of the abortus at the termination of pregnancy. If a previable abortus is then entered into research, it becomes the investigator's responsibility to observe those ethical research standards. These are stated in two parallel prohibitions: "If the [attending] physician determines that the fetus is not viable, it is not acceptable [for the researcher] [1] to maintain heart beat or respiration artificially in the abortus for the purpose of research. [2] Experimental procedures which of themselves will terminate respiration and heart beat may not be undertaken."

A third prohibition is tucked away in a statement of the system of "checks and balances" often invoked to suppress conflicts of interest in medical matters. "In order to insure that research considerations do not influence decisions as to timing, method, or extent of a procedure to terminate pregnancy," the NIH policy reads, "no investigator engaged in the research on the abortus may take part in these decisions. These are decisions to be made by the woman and her physician." If the requirement that no alteration be made in the timing, method, or extent of an abortion procedure is effective and seen to be effective in controlling practice that would be sufficient to quiet suspicion about the timing of the series of abortions from 11 to 30 days after injecting the women with rubella-vaccine virus in the case mentioned above.[2]

A clearly stated and assuredly observed prohibition of any changes made for research purposes in the timing, method, or extent of an abortion procedure seems clearly needed if the public is to *know,* for example, that the benefits to come from the antibiotic experiments reported in 1973,[3] which required hysterotomy, did not affect the choice of that method of abortion for those women in Boston City Hospital. Such a rule, if it had been in effect and was *perceived* to be assiduously observed and enforced by the profession, would forestall any questions raised by this article, which reports antibiotic experiments on women 15 to 43 years old and 10 to 20 weeks pregnant. Hysterotomy was performed on all the patients who received a single dose (14 women) and on 9 out of 17 who received multiple (4 to 20) doses. To know whether there was anything wrong with that (which we do not know), one would have to know the normal frequency of hysterotomies in that hospital, since there are three methods within the prudent choice of physicians after 13 weeks: hysterotomy (which imitates delivery by Caesarian section), saline injection, and prostaglandin injection (these two induce contractions imitative of vaginal delivery). But to know that nothing wrong was done in these experiments requires the proposed "guideline." Since it is not in force, we do not know, and doctors are in a quandary. Physician-researchers should, therefore, be the first to call for such a rule or regulation, if they mean not only to do right but to be seen always to do so.

If, on the contrary, physician-researchers feel somehow specially singled out or accused by the requirement that they never select the method or time of abortion because of research interests, then they need to acknowledge that if we do not have good fetal politics we will have bad fetal politics. Deeper than that, physician-researchers who may sometimes want to be free of regulation by an ethics consonant with that of the human community they serve may need to ponder the function of a code in any moral practice. "As a stream cannot rise above its source, so a code cannot change a low-grade man into a high-grade doctor, but it can help a good man to be a better man and a more enlightened doctor. It can quicken and inform a conscience, but not create one."⁴ A code, a guideline, an assuredly practiced and enforceable requirement is designed to help us live at our best under pressure (in this case, from the imperatives of research benefits).

Still I judge that the prohibition of any change in the time, method, or extent of abortion for the sake of medical experimentation was not the heart of the proposed NIH policy in regard to abortus research. That was rather the two prohibitions based on life signs, numbered in the text above. While "the possibility that the lungs can be inflated" is necessary to constitute viability, heartbeat remains a sign of life distinguishing a live abortus from a dead one. The NIH proposed policy's definitional reticence led to the avoidance of the term, "live" abortus. Still these two guidelines complete that definition. No research procedure may of itself terminate heartbeat or respiration. That means that these dying subjects—or in cases of abortion, these *condemned* ones—are to be allowed to complete their own dying and to die all the way without direct interventions. They are not to be hastened toward death for the purpose, or as a means, of studying them while dying.

On the other hand, no research procedure may be used that maintains heartbeat or respiration artificially in an abortus. That means that these dying or condemned fetal human beings are not to have their dying prolonged *in order* to study them. To that extent one keeps his distance from the dying; one does not make them simply means by which to obtain useful knowledge.

Of course, it is not for a moralist to say what sorts of beneficial research would be ruled out and what kinds remain permissible under these requirements. Certainly, not all fetal or abortus studies are excluded. While the foregoing ethical requirements "distance" research from tampering with the dying *process,* they do not, however, respectfully distance from *the dying* or allow only relevant therapeutic investigations upon them. Some of us may still believe that these dying ones ought also surely to be encompassed within the full extent of the protections expressed by Hans Jonas. Precisely because, here especially, we do not know the borderline between life and death, perhaps we should apply the "inflexible principle that utter helplessness demands utter protection." The small patient should be let die all the way, through the gamut of all definitions, and not be submitted to the ultimate violation of irrelevant, nontherapeutic research.[5] I think Jonas did not quite mean all definitions of death, e.g. cellular death (or if he did, he ought not to have meant that). Some of us may therefore believe that the not-dead, still living but dying fetal human being ought not to be submitted to irrelevant studies on the excuse that the experimental procedures *of themselves* do not directly extend, weaken, or terminate its vital signs.

It is important to note, however, that these ethical research requirements entail a more complete understanding of this novel potential research subject than would be provided by the regulation guiding physician judgment to the safe side of salvageability, standing alone. Here we have a subject who is neither a "dead fetus" (which was classed with macerated fetal material) nor yet even potentially a living infant. The difference between a dead and living abortus is not the same as the difference between a previable fetus and a viable baby. So also the Peel Report describes this subject as showing "some but not all signs of life" (not hesitating to say "life"); it was not content with measuring viability alone.

Thus we can tell life from death clearly enough to devise protections for this new subject of experimentation. The understanding that there is an alive human being long before viability sustains, and that alone can sustain, the issuance of protective ethical standards for this sort of research. We do *not* say that fetal research is "animal work" or human tissue study or investigations of the dead or of those in no way alive and no longer claiming the protection of the surrounding human community. Not only must the abortuses we are talking about be "living" in some *scientific* sense for anything to be learned unique from doing research on them. It is also the case that they must be already and still living in some *morally* relevant sense if such strong regulations have any meaning as distinct from rules governing the disposal of cadavers, for example. Far from abortion settling the question of fetal research, it could be that sober reflection on the use of the human fetus in research could unsettle the abortion issue.

Chapter 8

Controversial Cases

Meanwhile back at the vacuum in American medical public policy, our gathering public debate became increasingly acrimonious. Science writers report newsworthy cases, with the backing of quotations from leading physicians, as if the use of "fetal tissue" was the sole issue, and medical progress the sole source of medical ethics. "Pro-life" people mirror that mistake: they often seem to believe that research on fetal tissue is as outrageous as research on whole living fetal human being would be to them. Liberal intellectuals, for whom anti-Catholicism is still the acceptable anti-Semitism, complain that opposition to fetal research is only an attempt to arouse public feeling out of rancor over the lost cause of abortion control. Both extremes are in the wrong. Still, a policy vacuum in which prevailing community standards are frustrated from intruding upon the definition of the ethical limits of biomedical research is a good gathering place for rancor, deception, and self-deception. Assuredly, there is a public interest in determining across whose still living bodies we in future mean to be healed.

In the absence of clearly stated, publicly approved and enforceable guidelines, two legal prosecutions were begun recently in Boston. It is decidedly not edifying to read the discussion of these cases in our daily press or in medical journals; but it may be helpful if we apply to those two cases the standards promulgated in the Peel Report and in the proposed NIH guidelines.

On June 7, 1973, the *New England Journal of Medicine* published an article (mentioned above in connection with hysterotomies), reporting the findings from research at Boston City Hospital into whether certain antibiotics pass across the placental barrier into fetal blood or organs.[1] Early in 1974 five Boston physicians involved in that research were arrested under an 1814 grave-robbing statute and charged with "violation of sepulcher." From the published account of their research, it seems that it might have been forbidden had the NIH proposed guidelines been in force, since that statement categorically forbids any experimental procedures entailing risk to the fetus in situ undertaken in anticipation of abortion. Such would have been the application to this case if we invoke the fact (which in other connections physicians never weary of asserting to be a fact) that any medical intervention entails some risks. On the other hand, the research might not have been forbidden under the NIH ruling, since the antibiotics could, arguably, only have been benign to the fetus. Indeed, it could be argued that the administration of the antibiotic *might* factually benefit the fetus whose abortion was planned by protecting it from infection, in case its gestational age was miscalculated and it proved to be viable.

The Peel Report is clear: It forbids the administration of any drugs or carrying out any procedures during pregnancy "with the deliberate intent of ascertaining the harm that these might do to the fetus." The Boston physicians had no such intention. They were not testing for harm from placental passage —quite the contrary. Their objective in testing whether the two antibiotics would cross the placental barrier, and which would do so more efficiently, was to discover a way of protecting or treating the fetus at risk of infections, such as syphilis, in cases in which the pregnant women's allergy to penicillin precluded its use. These physicians were not testing drugs to ascertain their harm to the fetus across the placental barrier.

When the District Attorney broadened his investigation, two 24-week-old fetuses were discovered in the pathology department with no death certificates. Subsequently, Dr. Kenneth Edelin, chief resident in Ob-Gyn, was arrested for manslaughter of one of these fetuses, described as a "baby boy." The manner and means of his death is not known to the public, so we have no way of knowing the details of the charges that will be brought against Dr. Edelin nor how substantial (or insubstantial) the testimony against him will be. He should, of course, be presumed innocent until proven guilty. In the absence of more details we cannot tell exactly how to view the case in the light of the British and the American guidelines. The child may have been born or aborted *dead,* and then taken to the pathology department for studies. Then some far lesser offense could alone be charged.[2]

To construe a case, let us assume that a 24-week-old fetus is born or aborted intact and still living. Clearly, under the Peel ruling he could never have been taken to pathology for nontherapeutic studies, since the British guidelines *define* viability for research purposes at 20 weeks' gestational age, and they declare that when the fetus is viable after delivery a physician has "the ethical obligation to sustain its life so far as possible and it is both immoral and illegal to carry out any experiments on it which are inconsistent with treatment necessary to promote its life."

How the case would fare under the proposed American guidelines is less clear. The NIH notice, as we have seen, stipulates no age or other measurements on the safe side of viability. But it does require that "if there is a reasonable possibility that the life of the fetus may be saved, experimental and established methods may be used to achieve that goal." That, we have seen, allows the physician discretion in the matter of determining potential viability and the indicated treatment, even if it does mean to lay down the general standard, "treat all viable or potentially viable fetuses alike, regardless of the circumstances of their delivery" (as Walters contends). Therefore the physician's moral guilt depends very much on the circumstances of the case—beginning with whether this was a live-born fetus or not.

The thing that is insufferable is the absence of publicly approved standards. In that vacuum, and from reading the medical journals, one wonders what the research community would want the people's representative, a public prosecutor, to do if he is not on occasion—this or some other—to charge "manslaughter" or "violation of sepulcher."

An impartial reader must surely judge the editorials and articles in some medical journals commenting on the Boston cases to be as distraught and emotional as a "pro-life" spokesman's outrage over the use of fetal tissue or intact dead fetuses in research. Often their language reaches the same extremes. Thus in an editorial entitled "It's a Nightmare"—beginning with the word "Horrendous," *Medical Tribune,* June 5, 1974, took the position that "this attack upon physicians openly engaged in medical research under protocols subject to the approval of a committee of peers in a major hospital is *a violation of humanity . . .* this is no time for zealotry in *persecuting* physicians" (italics added). While correctly reporting the nature and importance of the antibiotic tests, it used diversionary tactics when it protested that "physicians should not be victimized as campaign issues," by prosecutors beholden to politicians in a state with a large Roman Catholic population; not beholden, the editorial seemed to imply, to protect human life at the borderline. "It's a very sad commentary," Assistant District Attorney Newman Flanagan replied, "that anyone would believe that a doctor was charged with manslaughter for the furtherance of political aims."[3] Moreover, by speaking of the "chilling effect on research utilizing fetal tissue"—and how without that we would not have developed polio vaccine—the *Medical Tribune* editorial entirely obfuscated the issue (like the most thoughtless "pro-lifer").

The tone of Barbara Culliton's article in *Science*[4] was similar to the *Medical Tribune's* editorial, although less pugalistic, more sad. She gives us a detail, however, that (if reported correctly) should either blunt the edge of any "scientific" criticism of "pro-lifers" who are supposed to have caused the uproar in Boston or else indicates a possible legal defense of these doctors. Each of the women gave written consent to their participation in the experiment. But Assistant District Attorney Newman Flanagan is quoted as saying that if the researchers had asked each of the women for consent to perform what amounts to the legal equivalent of an autopsy on her dead, aborted fetus, there would be no case.

Then to what did the women consent? Did they simply agree to take one of a variety of doses of either erythromycin or clindamycin and to let the doctors take blood samples *from them*? If that was all they agreed to, surely they did not validly consent to the whole course of the experimental procedure. If, however, they expressly agreed to the entire course of the procedure—from injection to studying the abortus' tissue—then Flanagan has no case. Is "consent to an injection" in cases such as this standard research practice?

Many scientists have too readily assumed that the Supreme Court's abortion decision settled the questions these cases raise, and further that it decreed the legal unprotectability of fetuses under investigations before or after abortion. A moment's reflection could have shown that here we have a gap, not a law. Into that gap flowed these cases and an acrimonious debate. I think it is unfair and a little dishonest to lay the responsibility for this totally at the door of embittered abortion foes.

Gaylin and Lappé write, for example, that "the Supreme Court absolved itself of any legal obligation . . . probably even to oversee experimentation for the first 6 months of fetal life. . . . the highest Court in the land probably did open the door to all and any experimentation in the first and second trimester of the fetus . . ."[5] They should know better. They should know that when the Court "absolved itself of any legal obligation to protect the life of the early fetus," there was another constitutional right alleged and in contest. There is no constitutional right to the benefits of medical progress. It is very poor legal interpretation to conclude that even a validly consenting women has now a quasi-constitutional right to deliver the fetus into the hands of a researcher.

In the abortion cases where state legislation prohibited that medical service, the woman's right to privacy was invoked against those laws. The situation is likely to be quite different in the case of state legislation banning fetal research. By what constitutional right is the woman to say that she should have the freedom to cause research to be done on her fetus? It was for this reason, I judge, that Reback concluded, "At a minimum, American researchers should understand that they face a legislative ban on experimentation unless a compromise solution is adopted."[6]

In any case, a correct characterization of our present situation is that some researchers seem to believe they can ride fetal research to total victory through the door of the Court's abortion decision. But at that threshold they meet again the foes of abortion. Research first stepped through, without waiting for a searching or adequate public or professionwide discussion of the moral issues. Each side accuses the other of bad faith. Each is guilty—of advocacy.

Perhaps we have bad fetal politics because we have not

found the way to invoke proper, widespread, and civil debate about this important issue of public and medical morality. A searching inquiry into the morality of fetal research must be the foundation of fetal politics, if it is to be good politics. A decision whether fetal research should be permitted or banned, severely limited or more generously allowed, should be the conclusion of a long and careful line of reasoning about it, and not a position taken at the beginning of the debate. To calm tempers, consider the following statement:

FETAL EXPERIMENTATION: Proper concern for the rights of the unborn child need not bring medical research to a halt. New therapeutic techniques can be used with the hope of proving them superior to traditional methods of treatment, after adequate theoretical work and animal experimentation has been carried out. Parents can give consent for experimental therapeutic treatment of the unborn if there is valid reason to believe that such treatment is in the best interests of the child. In addition, organs may be transplanted from the dead fetus, and tissue cultures may be developed from fetuses which are clinically judged to be dead according to the same criteria which would be used for a born child or adult. We recommend careful retrospective clinical and statistical study of defective babies for identification of teratogenic drugs. However, this is not the same thing as purposefully introducing known or suspected harmful substances for research purposes into the live unborn child or his mother which could cross the placental barrier. Systematic benefit should not be derived from systematic induced abortion. We do not approve of experiments which would be judged "cruel" or "senseless" by the average sensitive layman. And parents cannot consent to nontherapeutic research on unborn children who are being purposely aborted.

Now, that may not be enough to say. The statement, however, does make contact with the same tradition of medical ethics within which the medical community stands when trying to formulate guidelines governing fetal research. An unbiased reader will, I think, say that this is so. I would go further and say that it is a good place to begin, at least a better place to begin than with the final revision of the NIH guidelines, which we analyse in the following chapter. The statement was made by the Executive Director of the newly formed American Citizens Concerned for Life, Inc., before the Senate Subcommittee on Constitutional Amendments, August 21, 1974.

Chapter 9

The Revised Guidelines

On August 23, 1974, the Secretary of Health, Education, and Welfare published in the *Federal Register*[1] a revision of the November 16, 1973, proposed policy for the "Protection of Human Subjects." Since meanwhile the Congress had intervened, this was not an authoritative promulgation of regulations. Noting that both houses of Congress had reached agreement on, and the president had signed into law the National Research Act, the Secretary stated that his purpose in issuing a revised "notice of proposed rulemaking" was "to continue the public dialogue" begun by the original notice, to "assist the Department to develop final regulations," and to "also be available to the [national] Commission [for the Protection of Human Subjects in Biomedical and Behavioral Research] for their use during the course of their deliberations over the next two years."

The revision was made in the light of 450 responses to the first public notice. These responses came "largely from grantee and contractor organizations." That certainly shows that little "public dialogue" had been called forth by the administrative rule-making process. It can also be said that by the revisions introduced, the "research imperative" gained over the protections originally proposed. Whether one deems this to be a strengthening or a weakening of the regulations, it is important for us to pay attention to the changes, particularly in regard to research using the fetal human being.

The majority of the more than 400 letters received on research with children, born and unborn, touched on one or more aspects of research with fetuses, abortuses, and pregnant women. The department announced its rejection of the viewpoint of a "large number" of respondents who "disagreed entirely with the idea of permitting research with the fetus . . . or with the pregnant woman if the research might conceivably endanger the fetus." Because "differences in species" is so great,

75

reliance cannot be placed on research findings from work on animals alone. In addition, "the fetus and the newborn are not small adults"; they suffer from some diseases not encountered in adults, and they react differently to mankind's common illnesses and to similar treatments (e.g. drugs).

Many recommendations were received concerning the definition of viability.

> Some respondents suggested specific criteria such as birth weight, crown-rump length, or gestational age, similar to those used in England, such criteria to be reviewed and reissued periodically by the Department. . . . Some respondents urged that presence of fetal heart beat be definitive (whether or not there is respiration) while others urged that identifiable cortical activity be specified as an alternative sign of viability. Others objected strenuously to any distinctions as to the nature of fetal life, holding that the physician's obligation should be the same to any fetus regardless of weight, size, or age of gestation.[2]

Here again, the department held to its original (1973) position. "The issue of viability is a function of technological advance," it stated, "and therefore must be decided with reference to the medical realities of the present time. . . . Heartbeat and respiration are, jointly, to be the indicators of viability," since "current technology is such that a fetus, given the benefit of available medical therapy, cannot survive unless the lungs can be inflated so that respiration can take place." Within this understanding of viability as a variable dependent on medical technology, the department expressed in no uncertain terms the medical obligation to save all salvageable lives at any time to come: "In the future, if technology has advanced to the point of sustaining a fetus with noninflatable lungs, the definition can and should be modified."

It is difficult to understand the Department's rejection of the specification in terms of birth weight, crown-rump length, or gestational age. Those who have some reason to object to that are the respondents who held a physician's obligation to be the same to any fetus regardless of weight, size, or age of gestation. Other physicians and researchers should be the first to urge the protection of the fetus (and at the same time of themselves) in those terms safely short of viability. Even those who hold that a physician's obligation to the fetus is continuous ought to agree, provided the parameters thus defined are accompanied by other adequate regulations. A good case can be made, for example, on behalf of such measurable distinctions between abortuses that are ineligible and those eligible for research in the context of *other regulations* that go on to distinguish permissible and impermissible research. To define pre-viability for research purposes need not mean that then all is permitted. We need such a definition even if we go on to say that ethical research ought never to extend or directly terminate vital signs, or ought not be done to ascertain harm to the fetus, or ought not to be done if there is any discernible risk.

However, Secretary Weinberger stated that, while the distinction between a viable and nonviable fetus is meaningful, "the Department does not believe that the use of weight, size, gestational age and/or cortical activity is a valid substitute for the judgment of a physician."

Perhaps so, if the issue is viability in general. Of course, the fetus is viable at all stages unless it is removed from its natural environment. In face of that actual viability at all stages of development, in abortion practice we define viability in another, artificial way. In the matter of research practice we need another, more or less artificial, definition of viability: viability for research purposes. It seems to me that researchers, if they have any regard for values beyond the research imperative, should be the first to insist that eligible abortuses in medical experiments be defined safely short of *possibly* viable birth weight, crown-rump length, and gestational age. They, of all people, should want to be seen to do right. Those dimensions constitute an *outer limit* on the safe side of viability (to be updated with future progress in medical technology). Those dimensions also are only the beginning of a proper analysis of ethical practice in fetal research. As that analysis proceeds, some sorts of experimentation ought surely to be excluded, perhaps many research designs may prove incompatible with protections due the fetus, perhaps all experimentation should be forbidden on these other grounds except for controlled observations or interven-

tions foreseen to bear no risk of harm. But none of these up-
shots are grounds for not defining what we are talking about
using in research.

Of course, we can understand those who insist that heartbeat
or identifiable cortical activity should be signs of life claiming
our utmost protection and that such lives should be excluded
from nonbeneficial medical experimentation. We can understand the views of those who say that no distinctions should be
made on account of any weight, age, or size; and I am inclined
to agree with them if that alone limits our obligation to protect
from harm. What is utterly incomprehensible is that the secretary of HEW should deem no compromise to be worthy, that
he would prefer to have medical researchers possibly experimenting on "viable" babies (in the current meaning of that
expression) rather than endorse standards assuring the public
that at least such experimentation would not take place. This is
a simple matter: the point is not the meaning of viability for
the purpose of decisions promoting the saving of life or allowing
to die in the practice of fetal medicine and pediatrics. On that,
doubtless there is no "valid substitute for the judgment of a
physician." The point is rather a limitation upon the definition
of viability for research purposes; and here surely there is a
need to give direction to the judgment of the researcher. I do
not say that *below* stated birth weight, crown-rump length, or
gestational age abortus research is justified. I do say that we
need measurable limits *beyond which* it clearly is not.

Now we have to consider the startling revisions made on
the guidelines as proposed in 1973.

THE FETUS IN UTERO

The categorical prohibition of experimentation entailing
risk to the fetus in anticipation of abortion was in the 1974
document radically modified. The proposed policy now reads:
"No activity . . . involving fetuses *in utero* or pregnant women,
may be undertaken unless (1) the purpose of the activity is
to benefit the fetus or to respond to the health needs of the
mother, or (2) the activity [is] conducted as part of (but
not prior to the commencement of) a procedure to terminate

the pregnancy and is for the purpose of evaluating or improving methods of prenatal diagnosis, methods of prevention of premature birth, or methods of intervention to offset the effects of genetic abnormality or congenital injury."

The first of the above provisions results from a decision to consider the fetus in utero in a larger context than planned abortion. There can, of course, be no ethical objection to the therapeutic investigations this provision describes. However, it also entails the removal of the strong affirmations of a medical obligation "to protect the developing fetus from avoidable harm" and the warning not to compromise medicine's respect for the dignity of human life by taking into account an individual's "expectation of life." Those statements were removed in shifting consideration of the fetus in utero from the limited context of planned abortion.

The second provision speaks to that context where those affirmations are needed. Several respondents had urged that the purposes of research on the fetus in utero should alone be deemed a sufficient ethical justification if abortion was in view. The comments apparently included improving methods of abortion and birth control among their justifying research aims. These were not accepted by the department, whose reasons may all be described as aiming to improve the medical care of children, born or unborn. It can be argued, however, as we have seen, that if we are going to approve experimentation on these dying, condemned ones, there is something to be said for the relevance of research directed to improving methods of abortion (from which they are dying) in contrast to, to them, entirely irrelevant investigations.

The department did not agree that a good purpose was sufficient grounds to justify fetal research. It added the stipulation that such research can be permitted not simply in anticipation of abortion, but "only when done as part of a procedure properly performed to terminate a pregnancy." The department has chosen "to permit research to be undertaken *from which there will be risk of harm to the fetus* if such research is conducted as part of the abortion procedure" (italics added).

This amounts to a sweeping reversal of the original draft. The department has now "tentatively concluded that consideration of risk vs. benefit with respect to fetal research does not seem to be appropriate." In November, 1973, the view was that the fetus should be protected from every avoidable harm, that age, condition, or life-expectancy ought not to compromise our respect for the dignity of life or its protection. Now potentially harmful research with the fetus in utero would be permitted, if it is a part of the abortion procedure itself. Except for the latter reservation, the DHEW-NIH guideline concerning harmful research amounts to a retreat to the position expressed more vividly by Dr. Kurt Hirschhorn in the original *Post* article, or to the view of other apologists who believe that abortion means that there are no moral limits upon what research may do stemming from risks or harm to the fetal human being itself.

"It is not intended that this provision be construed to permit fetal research in anticipation of abortion prior to the commencement of the termination procedure itself." That means that the woman's consent and her right to change her mind (which fades by the time of the abortion) have been made the sole operative considerations putting limits upon socially beneficial research on the fetus in utero. In the original paragraph, a woman's right to change her mind about the abortion worked jointly with, if not subordinate to, medicine's obligation to do no harm—to forbid placing the fetus in utero under additional experimental risks. Fetal research in anticipation of abortion is still forbidden. But that means "anticipation earlier on." Once the procedure to terminate pregnancy has begun, research can proceed without regard for the fetal subject.

It is true there may have been an unmentioned reason for the original prohibition of risky research in anticipation of abortion, namely, the frequency of miscalculation of gestational age by one month. If that had been the case, and the fetus happened to be "delivered" alive, an experiment that had been begun might injure it. This consideration lends support to the department's original position and obliquely to its present one; but that is nowhere mentioned. That also is the reason the use of gestational age in determining eligibility for research ought to be fixed more than one month below possible viability, in the context of current and future ability of medicine to save the newborn—if in our abortion practice we already have not stepped across that line and are sometimes aborting viable babies *and mean to use them also in fetal research.*

In a "correction" issued on October 21, 1974,[3] Secretary Weinberger deleted the paragraph containing the strongest statements quoted above. That is, the affirmative sentence "The Department has provisionally chosen . . . to permit research to be undertaken from which there will be risk of harm to the fetus if such research is conducted as part of the abortion procedure" was taken out. The secretary stated in his October correction that that sentence "incorrectly implies that, under the proposed rule-making, fetuses for which abortion is contemplated may be placed at greater risk than fetuses in general." But that refers to another matter, namely, the categorical ban on fetal research begun "prior to the commencement of the termination procedure itself" (a sentence also in the deleted paragraph). The paragraph as a whole seems to me simply to repeat with no substantial change what is said in a previous paragraph that was retained. Weinberger repeats essentially the same judgment in his "correction": "the proposed rule making bans the undertaking of research . . . involving the fetus prior to the commencement of the abortion procedure, at which point the question of risk to the fetus is no longer at issue." Only the bald statement about research doing possible harm was removed. That statement seemed too candid. The position is the same with the correction.

It is clear what the department means by "not prior to the commencement of" a procedure to terminate pregnancy. Research genuinely a part of the abortion procedure would seem to be reduced to controlled observation or study of that procedure, altered in no respect. Research during the time of the abortion procedure could, by contrast, introduce limited or unlimited alterations of that procedure or at least introduce parallel actions not required by or normally part of an abortion: only these would yield significant research benefits. While it stretches the ordinary meaning of "part," I take the department to mean research simply coincident in time with the abortion. Otherwise, there would be no intervention to constitute the investigation; only "controlled observation." Then why speak of risk or harm from "part" of the abortion procedure?

If that is correct, the 1974 version of "Protection of Human Subjects" has introduced a type of fetal research on which the original 1973 version was silent, namely, what was above called Type (2) research, at about the time of abortion (adding that then harm or pain to the fetus is removed from ethical consideration), in contrast to research on the fetus in utero in anticipation of an abortion a day or several days in the future, and in contrast also to live abortus research. Furthermore, it is significant to note that research "at the time" or "as a part" of an abortion procedure was categorically forbidden by the Peel Report. At least this seems to be the British regulation on one reading of a condition governing use of the whole dead fetus or fetal tissue, that "dissection of the dead fetus *or experiments on the fetus* or fetal material do not occur in the operating theatre or place of delivery" (italics added). Concerning the present DHEW-NIH permission of fetal experimentation in the place of delivery or abortion, the question to be asked is how many valid consents from women can be secured to such activities under those circumstances.

The provision in the American regulations for research at risk of possible harm to the fetus in utero at the time or as part of the abortion procedure is still severely circumscribed by the rule that anyone engaged in such research "will have no part in: (1) any decisions as to the timing, method, or procedures used to terminate the pregnancy, and (2) determining the viability of the fetus at the time of the pregnancy." The first stipulation, if adhered to, raises the questions how, then, research can possibly be made a "part" of the abortion procedure and how a knowing, i.e. foreknowing, consent could be secured.

LIVE ABORTUS RESEARCH

Significant modifications were also made in the proposed regulations governing research with the still living, previable abortus. Before, the use of the dying fetus could not involve experimental procedures that either directly terminate or artificially maintain or prolong its vital signs. The fetal human being, while under medical investigation, was to be allowed to complete its own dying. Now, only one of these two provisions remains: "Experimental procedures which would terminate the heartbeat or respiration of the abortus will not be employed." (Why respiration?, we may ask, in view of the cruciality of respiration in defining viability? At that point, where there is respiration, have we not been told that every effort should be made to save the infant's life and no experiments are permitted?)

With regard to the other provision, it is now allowed that the fetal subject may conditionally be withheld from death so that research may gain: "Vital functions of an abortus will not be artificially maintained," the 1974 policy reads, "except where the purpose of the activity is to develop new methods for enabling the abortus to survive to the point of viability." We are not told for how long a time these justifying reasons would warrant artificially maintaining vital functions in a living fetus, and thus interfering with its dying. One or two hours? A day or two? A month or two? Indefinitely? If the idea is that procedures which aim to develop rescue techniques should be stopped, in the case of a particular fetal subject of experiment, safely before it seems likely to succeed, then we are back at the profound moral paradox that the closer this sort of abortus research comes to proving to have treatment value in a particular case, the more continuation should be condemned. Surely, ethics must insist that the closer a rescue procedure approaches success, the stronger the fetal subject claims our effort to save it.

The department's present position was a compromise between those respondents who argued that termination of heartbeat ought not to be prohibited, since that could prove essential in developing certain surgical techniques, on the one hand, and on the other those who simply urged that the maintenance of vital functions and signs ought to be allowed for research purposes other than for developing rescue techniques. The department rejected the former; and, in accepting the latter position, it called its radical revision of the 1973 proposals a mere "expansion." In doing so, however, it rightly emphasized again the gulf that separates research with a dead abortus or fetal tissue from research with "the whole fetus or abortus, functioning as an organism with detectable vital signs."

In conclusion, there are three notable instances of a more general character repeated throughout the revised document, which clearly indicate that the research imperative wins in its contest with the protection of human subjects.

The first seems minor at first glance. "Consent committees" are to be established to monitor the obtaining of valid consents, the conduct of specific research, the withdrawal of subjects, etc. That could prove a major protection. But then an exception is allowed by the following provision. (I quote from the case of fetal human research subjects, where the exception seems not to be applicable, since risk of harm was deemed irrelevant to research that is part of an abortion procedure.) :

> Where a particular activity, involving fetuses *in utero* or pregnant women, presents negligible risk to the fetus, an applicant or offerer may request the secretary to modify or waive the requirement in paragraph (a) of this section [the consent committees]. If the secretary finds that the risk is indeed negligible and other adequate controls are provided, he may (with the advice of the Ethical Advisory Board) grant the request in whole or in part.

That loophole may be defensible because it limits some of the complexity in the rather cumbersome administrative procedures and committee structures envisioned by the proposal. However, it raises some fundamental questions. If, as seems likely, the "exception" is designed to allow placing the fetus in utero at risk if the risk is deemed negligible, has it not reintroduced the whole class of experimentations on the fetus in utero in anticipation of abortion—meaning anticipation earlier on than the time of, or as a part of, the termination procedure itself? After all, the question of risk or harm was declared irrelevant to the in utero research permitted by this revision because it is part of an abortion procedure. Then what sort of research may the secretary admit by making an exception, if it is not experimentation on the fetus in utero in advance of an abortion—provided the risk of harm is deemed negligible? Then do we not have here, in effect, an endorsement of both Type (1) and Type (2) research, the former brought back in as an "exception-making" procedure? That seems a subterfuge to legitimate both risky and harmful fetal research with little or no argument for either, and without going public in the formulation of fetal research policy. I believe that we need a further "correction" of these revised guidelines that will tell us that the "exception" paragraph has incorrectly been taken to imply that the secretary means to approve research on "fetuses for which abortion is contemplated" that will place them "at greater risk than fetuses in general." The exceptions put in jeopardy much more than the consent requirement.

The second provides for the modification of these consent procedures in the case of fetal research done abroad.

> Activities ... to be conducted outside the United States are subject to the requirements of this subpart, except that the consent procedures specified herein may be modified if it is shown to the satisfaction of the Secretary that such procedures, as modified, are acceptable under the laws and regulations of the country in which the activities are to be performed.

To that it is a proper ethical response to say that a human subject is a human subject in need of protection whether he (she, or it) is a South American, an African, as Asian, a Scandinavian no less than if he (she, or it) is a North American. What is right and needed for one is right and needed by the other. And it is a proper political response to say that the implication of the American taxpayer in overbearing research done abroad is no less offensive than if this is done within the borders of the United States. Would we say, for example, that research done abroad on prisoners should be funded by the federal government if the secretary certifies that the procedures satisfy the laws and regulations governing the treatment of prisoners in the country in which the research is done? The DHEW-NIH proposed guidelines allow that exception, too. If that is the way the people of the United States mean in future to be healed, then medical progress, too, is imperialistic. Do we really mean to say that American researchers should do unto others as we would not want done unto us?

In the third and final instance, the proposed policy opens futuristic doors by its definitions that are descriptions of remote scientific possibilities while it assiduously confines its protective regulations to close-at-hand possibilities by the definitions that are regulative. For example, " '*In vitro* fertilization' means any fertilization of the human ova which occurs outside the body of a female, either through admixture of donor sperm and ova or by any other means." Both "donor ova" and "by any other means" open vistas not covered by the regulations. An example of the strict limitation imposed upon the rule-making process is the department's rejection of those comments proposing that "pregnancy" be defined to begin at fertilization. "While the Department has no argument with the conceptual definition as proposed above, it sees no way of basing regulations on the concept. Rather in order to provide an administerable policy, the definition must be based on existing medical technology which permits confirmation of pregnancy." I think there can be no quarrel with that reasoning, except that then the department ought not to have opened inviting doors in its scientific descriptions for which it proposed no regulation, as in the "definition" of in vitro fertilization above.

A final illustration brings us back to our main topic. The department's "intent" in the definition of "fetus" was that this be construed to encompass both the product of in vivo conception and the product of in vitro fertilization which is subsequently "implanted in the donor of the ovum." So far, so good. But then our attention is called to the fact that "it is only with respect to the protections available to the non-implanted product of *in vitro* fertilization that the regulations are silent." The reason offered for that silence is that "given the state of research, we believe that such stipulation would be premature." Clearly, however, an abundant supply of embryonic and fetal human research subjects cultured in the laboratory is in prospect (not simply zygotes undergoing cleavage that may now be discarded while others are implanted). By its regulatory austerity, while pointing in other language to developments to come, the department insures that protective regulation shall always fall behind research. Lest experimentation be prematurely foreclosed, the department may have guaranteed instead that in the ever-receding future, there will always be human fetal research subjects that already *needed* protection.

The question of human research using the products of in vitro fertilization was again addressed in the "correction" on October 21, 1974. On that occasion the secretary simply said more elaborately what had been said before, in effect legitimating a new sort of human research under cover of providing procedures for regulating it.

> The Department has . . . concluded that while it is necessary to impose certain restraints, it is contrary to the interests of society to set permanent restrictions on research which are based on the successes and limitations of current technology. Therefore, the Department would expect the Ethical Advisory Board, which must review all applications involving *in vitro* fertilization (whether or not implantation is contemplated) to weigh, with respect to specific proposals, the state of the art, legal issues, community standards, and the availability of guidelines to govern each research situation. In sum, if there is a possibility that the conceptus might be sustained *in vitro* beyond the earliest stages of development, the Ethical Advisory Board is to consider this possibility, and determine what guidelines should govern decisions affecting that fetus, if the research is to be permitted. If, on the other hand, implantation is attempted and achieved, then regulations governing the fetus *in utero* shall apply.

When better loopholes are made, doubtless DHEW-NIH will make them.

Chapter 10

Who "Consents" to
Fetal Research?

We have seen several themes weaving in and out as we try
to think about ethical dimensions of the use of the human
fetus in research. Where this question and the abortion issue
coincide, great strain is placed on the meaning of the consent
requirement. Who "consents" for this new sort of research
subject? By whose authority is the fetus chosen or entered
into medical experimentation intended to be beneficial only
to others?

The easiest answer—because it has a familiar analogy in
research policy and practice—is to say that parents (or one
parent) can properly substitute their consent (or her consent)
for the consent of the abortus as research subject, just as
parents or guardians can substitute their consent for that of
an infant or small child—absent in both cases any capacity
in them to consent to become "normal volunteers." This is
the answer given by the NIH document, "Protection of Human
Subjects." Parental or maternal consent is required.

The Peel Report, however, equivocates. It firmly provides
that the mother have the opportunity to declare any special
wishes she may have about the disposal of a dead fetus resulting from an abortion. On the other hand, a live-born fetus
who subsequently dies is treated in English law like any other
deceased person; and also, generally in English law and medical ethical standards, no one can validly consent to submit an
infant (a live-born fetus, though he subsequently may die) to
medical trials except those related to promoting its life. Thus,
paradoxically, consent is called for in case of the disposal of a
dead fetus, while maternal consent is invalid to place a live-
born fetus into nontherapeutic research. The dilemma seems
to be: shall researchers obtain an expression of the wishes of
women about the disposal of their dead fetuses, in hope or

anticipation that the fetus may be alive at time of delivery (abortion), whose entrance as subjects into pure research no one's consent could then legitimate? Such quandaries result from a conceptual failure, perhaps an unavoidable one: the failure fully to *define* this new research subject falling between a dead intact abortus and a still-living, previable abortus. Does the latter merge with the former (where the woman's wishes are consulted) or with liveborn babies (where her consent is severely limited in British law, if not invalid except to promote their lives)? These are quandaries raised by the British guidelines.

Concerning a fetus "born" alive (whether by termination or not), which then dies—where registration of the deceased applies—the Peel Report requires that "enquiry must be made as to whether there is objection on the part of the parent before the body can be used for research."

Concerning a fetus "born dead" by termination, however, "there is no statutory requirement to obtain the parent's consent for research, but equally no statutory power to ignore the parent's wishes." Under those circumstances—where registration is not legally required—the report observes, "to seek consent would be an unnecessary source of distress to parents. We share this view but believe [and here the Report introduces its advocacy of a form of general or routine consent, or power to dissent] the parent must be offered the opportunity to declare any special directions about the disposal of the fetus."

There is finally a paragraph which states: "There are also areas of research which whilst not jeopardizing the health and welfare of the fetus are not of direct benefit to that particular fetus. In such cases we consider that express consent should be obtained from the parent." "Express consent" is needed, I take the report to mean, in two cases: (1) research involving the fetus in utero that is not dangerous, since only studying harm to the fetus was expressly forbidden whether the woman consents or not; and (2) research involving the still living abortus, since use of the dead fetus is covered by the provisions above. If this is correct, the Peel Report does not wrestle with the morality of terminating or extending vital signs in the living previable abortus, and instead covers that by the parent's *prior* express consent to research on her dead abortus—which happens, then, to be born alive but previable.

One can, of course, go in the British direction and argue that the analogy between the fetus and the infant behind the American guidelines' doctrine of consent justifies nothing, because parents have no moral right, in the first place, to enter their children into potentially harmful investigations intended only to be socially beneficial, or merely for the accumulation of knowledge. If parents have only the moral right to consent to therapeutic trials that are medically on behalf of their children, then on that ground alone a woman's consent to "pure" medical experimentation on her abortus would be stopped.

But let us not take that route, although it seems to me entirely sufficient. Instead of searching for analogy with experiments on children, let us rather search out the difference between these two cases and ask whether the fact of elective abortion does not enfeeble the analogy to the point of morally nullifying any extension of our current beliefs and practices (even if, as I believe, these are morally flawed) in regard to "proxy consent" in the case of children submitted to non-therapeutic research to this new class of research subjects.

The proposed NIH policy, "Protection of Human Subjects," takes the contrary view, as I have said; it gives the easiest answer, or at least the one ordinarily to be expected in our present context: "consent for abortion does not necessarily entail disinterest on the part of the pregnant woman in what happens to the product of conception." Since some women "feel strongly" while others do not feel strongly about what may, or may not, be done to the aborted fetus, every woman undergoing an abortion should be given "the opportunity to declare her wishes." Her consent to the "application of any research procedures to the aborted fetus" must be secured at the time of admission to the hospital.

I take that to mean more than signing a general consent form agreeing to simply "any" research. The NIH guidelines specifically state that "maternal consent" must be "freely given and based on full disclosure, each time approved research is conducted on an abortus." If the research protocol entailed studying the fetus if expelled whole, or studying the whole fetus with a heartbeat, or a living brain or other developing organs, that should be explained to her. Merely stating the requirement in this strong sense begins to raise questions whether a valid consent can be secured under those circumstances. Anyone who wanted to stop whole, live abortus research might consider endorsing this proposal, and insist that it be strictly observed and policed by ethical review boards. Moreover, is it not cruel to attempt to get a valid informed consent under those circumstances?

Going deeper still, one may object that the very meaning of legitimate proxy "consent" has been abrogated in the majority of contemporary abortion situations. Possessing the moral authority to consent is not a matter of strong or weak feelings. The fundamental model for legitimate parental consent in place of a child's is—as I indicated above—proxy consent that is medically *on behalf of* the child. In therapeutic investigations the child is construed to consent as if he were competent to do so. Building upon this foundation, American research policy and practice and the NIH guidelines, deem parental proxy consent to be valid in carefully circumscribed instances of non-beneficial research as well.

In all these cases parental consent is sought and is believed valid because parents are presumed to be "caretakers" for their infant children. Care is the attribute or virtue that qualifies parents as proxies, not strong or weak feelings, or strong or mild "interest"—certainly not for the sake of their own feelings or equanimity in the face of anything that may happen to their children or, in this instance, to the products of their conception. By using the expression "supplementary judgment" (appropriate enough in cases where *both* parental consent and the consent of an adolescent are sought) to describe also parental decisions to enter children below the "age of discretion" (seven years of age) into nonbeneficial medical experiments, the NIH policy in fact smooths the way for decisions to enter abortuses into research projects that do not depend on any remaining care in parenting.

Nevertheless, there are proscriptions elsewhere in this policy document that, if taken seriously as models, seem to go in the direction of invalidating a woman's consent to abortus research in at least many contemporary abortion decisions. This policy specifically disqualifies parental consent from having anything to do with entering into research children who are "detained in an institutional setting pursuant to a court order." It specifically and categorically states that "persons detained in a correctional facility while awaiting sentence, or in a hospital facility for presentencing diagnostic observation," are excluded from participation in research. (In response to the objection that persons in correctional institutions should not "be denied the benefits of innovative procedures, particularly those concerned with sociological research," the department modified this prohibition and in the August 1974 revision permits such research "when the risk is negligible and the intent of the activity is therapeutic for him or relates to the nature of his confinement.") Categorically excluded from participation in research involving risk are "children with no natural or adoptive parents available to participate in consent deliberations, and children detained by court order in a residential facility, whether or not natural or adoptive parents are available."

Are not these better models for the ethics of research involving abortuses than any of the models that even now stretch to the limit the "caretaking" presumption ascribed to parents? Are not captive populations of children who are excluded from research more analogous to the unborn in elective abortion decisions than children with responsible parents? Ought not medical practice or the government intervene to protect the condemned from further molestation in their dying, even as it is proposed to intervene to protect certain captive populations of children from the sovereign sway of parent or guardian consent? It would be odd if we do not rescue from the deputyship of parents abortuses who have been abandoned by them as we would children abandoned in institutions. Certainly this is the case, if we do not mean to abandon the cardinal medical ethical principle that "respect for the dignity of human life must not be compromised whatever the age, circumstance, or expectation of life of the individual," and if by any chance we still believe that measures for the "protection of children as subjects of biomedical research must be applied with equal rigor and with additional safeguards to the fetus."

The question is whether a woman by her abortion decision has not waived any claim to consent on behalf of, or render any supplementary judgments in behalf of, the abortus. This is not a matter of feelings, further anguish, or interests, however strong these appeals may be. It it rather a question of moral authority to decide—the competence to decide—concerning the risks, harm, or pain that may be inflicted on another life, even in the course of using it for social benefit. So far, such moral authority and responsibility require some relic of care or an actualized biology-based care, or at least a plausible pretense of it, that is rebuttable both in law and morals and which —even in the case of entering children into clearly nonbeneficial experiments upon them—can still be counted on to draw some outer limits if parents are actually informed what is to be done. That is to say, no other feeling than parental care is counted on either to validate or to limit proxy consent. The question then, in the present instance, is whether women undergoing elective abortion have or do not have a remaining claim to perform actions which care for the abortus and protect it from further indignity, neglect, pain, or harm. A strong case can be made that a woman—at least in many instances of abortion—has no standing to claim social endorsement of her moral authority to decide in cases of fetus or abortus research.

LeRoy Walters describes in the following way the "qualitative difference between the two types of consent" we have been discussing. In research on infants and children, parents consent for an individual for whom they know they will bear financial and social responsibility in the future. In research on a previable fetus in planned abortion, they would consent to research on an individual "which they are sure they will not be obliged to raise." Walters then lays down the following general stipulation: "This disanalogy" between the consent situations "could be overcome only if parents [or one parent] were willing to act *as if* the fetus would survive and later become their [or her] responsibility."[1]

Simply to state that requirement discloses the impossibility of any such expectation in validating proxy consent in many abortion situations—at least as a general rule upon which to base fetal research practice. Even so, I would say that Walters' formulation externalizes a possible future with that child (and does so self-referentially). That can serve to brace us to live up to only part of the real meaning of parenting. On a more interior view of parental proxy consent to abortus research, parents or the woman would have to be assumed able and willing to act *as if* she (they) *cared* for the fetus. Perhaps such an assumption could be "verified" in some or many cases, but that seems doubtful in a great number of cases.

As a general rule there should be good reason to suppose parents to be on the whole better qualified in the protection of these novel research subjects than other "candidates" for the "position" of initiator of fetal experimentation. In any case, the *as ifs* express the only conditions under which the disanalogy between the consent situations can be overcome.

Since we are exploring and not settling the issue at this point, perhaps we could say that a woman who underwent a "just and necessary" abortion, who except for the pressure of inexorable necessity threatening life or health would have endured great inconveniences and considerable suffering in order to keep and care for her child, might claim the deputyship of deciding whether her abortus should or should not be submitted to medical experiments. Perhaps she could legitimately consent to one sort of research while refusing another as degrading to the product of her conception. In such a case, I imagine that the last thing she would wish would be that her necessarily condemned child should as an abortus be further used. Perhaps I am wrong. Even so, surely it is morally outrageous—and many persons who countenance liberalized abortion believe it would be morally outrageous—to designate women who elect abortion for comparatively trivial reasons, or for social convenience or economic betterment, to the socially responsible role or ascribe to them the decisional competence and deputyship to say whether that abortus should or should not be used in medical experimentation. Anyone who believes that to be right must be able to tolerate a contradiction at the heart of his practical moral reasoning. If not a contradiction, he must simply believe consent for another rests on biology and not on responsibility.

The medical community needs someone at the point of entry into research with the authorization to dispose of live abortuses or of the fetus in situ. What is more natural than to light upon that person who at the outermost limits of the community of care for individual children traditionally has had authorization to consent on their behalf? Still it is a different role assignment. The authority to dispose of abortuses has one moral meaning; legitimate proxy consent has another. The former role seems destined to displace and replace the latter. The woman in abortion situations is, then, a convenient disposer of abortuses in initiating the process of socially beneficial medical experimentation. But that is a different deputyship. One is based on the right to privacy and individualistic decision; the other is based on a claim to care.

Moreover, we can think of other and morally less contradictory schemes to start the research process, if that is the objective. The attending physician has responsibility to declare the fetus viable or nonviable if it is expelled whole. He should save it (or "may" try to do so) even if the woman wanted to get rid of it. According to the NIH guidelines, he is not supposed to alter the time, method, or extent of his procedure in terminating the pregnancy under the influence of research considerations. Presumably he does not deliberately produce abortuses that are likely to be good research material. If to this extent he is a physician attending the fetus as well as the woman, why is he not a good candidate for the office of disposer of abortuses for research purposes, at least as legitimate in that role as women undergoing elective abortions?

Alternatively, it could be the practice at our medical centers that all previable abortuses be routinely used in medical research, unless the woman expressly and on her own initiative dissents. That would abolish the role of consent, or of a maternal disposer of abortuses, while systematically entering all abortuses into needed medical research unless the woman objected. The Peel Report in Great Britain, unlike its U.S. counterpart, went in this direction when it only required certification that "the mother has had opportunity to declare any special wishes about the disposal of the dead fetus." Doubtless the intention was to present the issue in those general terms, without any specific mention of fetal experimentation as a possibility. She might say in response that she did not care to know anything about it, or didn't care anyway—in which case the abortus would routinely be considered eligible for research purposes. Presumably, these requirements do not apply to the dead fetus. Or she could say she wanted it treated with tender loving care, not trashed in the incinerator, perhaps buried (whether *she* wanted to do this or not)—in which case, I suppose, her abortus could not be used in experimentation. Consulting her express wishes is required by the Peel Report only in the case of nonjeopardizing research on the fetus *in situ* and in case she had consented, and a previable abortus *happened* to be produced alive.

As a practical matter, we may ask whether (under the proposed U.S. scheme) the woman's signature on a consent form upon admission to the hospital may turn out to be the actual practice. If so, that would not mean much more than routinizing live abortus research, with an opening for her dissent, as for a dead abortus in the British system. Is it credible to believe that physicians intend adequately to inform her of the specific details of experiments in readiness for her abortus at the medical center in case it survives the abortion procedure? Indeed, would it be compassionate for them to do so?

Alexander Capron has, in the case of children, proposed another possibility that could be extended to aborted fetuses entered into nontherapeutic research.[2] He suggests "selection by guardian." That, he contends, would preserve "some of the intent of the informed consent system," namely the protection of the subject from undue or useless risk "in a manner similar to the one which he would himself have chosen." Selectors would end the "charade" of "substituted consent" which implies or construes "self-choice" on the part of the child. In most abortions today, substituted consent would, indeed, except in rare cases, be a charade in the case of the aborted fetus, if the woman or the erstwhile parents are designated to that post. Once we understand that selectors are guardians at the point of entrance into socially beneficial research (not surrogate parents caring for the child), then we would be free to consider other candidates for the disposition of fetuses who are as well or better qualified than women undergoing abortions.

Selectors, whether the attending physician or someone else not a member of the research team, could be used in some manner in combination with two other suggestions Capron makes for the advancement of nontherapeutic research using young subjects: selection on the basis of medical fitness for the experiment, and random selection. Thus, for example, selectors could first make judgments as to the nonviability and the protection of the fetus (e.g. from pain); he then could select for medical fitness for the study; and finally he could randomize among those medically fit in order to insure that no social, economic, or racial class of women having abortions are unequally made the providers of abortuses deemed necessary for research on prenatal development and diseases.

Random selection would have this further advantage: public discussion and debate would be needed to adopt it as a public policy. Parents or women of all races and classes, those in Tarrytown no less than welfare mothers, would (as participants in setting medical policy in the direction of abortus research) know that this would be a burden, if burden it is, that falls equally or randomly on all alike; and that we are not going to make medical progress again mainly across the bodies (or "products" of the bodies) of the poor and the black. A provision could be attached to such a system to give effect to a woman's dissent or "conscientious objection" to any such use of the product of her conception.

These alternative arrangements come to mind because it is such an extreme moral paradox to designate a woman who is planning a medically unnecessary abortion to be the one charged with consenting or not consenting "for" the abortus and with protecting it from further avoidable harm. It is worth repeating that her proxy consent never before was thought to express her "feelings" alone or the degree of her interest in a child (and now in an abortus entered into research), but rather her judgment concerning the interests of the fetus or child. That, I suggest, she has abandoned, except in those cases when the abortion decision was impelled by very weighty considerations. If the disposition of abortuses for research purposes is such an utterly different role, one can as a general rule readily think of other candidates for that office besides pregnant women.

The foregoing are thought experiments designed to highlight a crucial ethical issue in abortus research. On the other hand, one can perversely prefer the suggestion of the NIH policy statement, provided it is assiduously carried out, namely, that the possibility of a whole fetus being expelled be explained to pregnant women seeking an abortion, and the contemplated research explained to them, so that prior informed consent is validly secured. That may seem an inhuman thing to try to enlist on such an occasion, only rendered humane because it is not meant to be carried out, except by general consent forms signed thoughtlessly by pregnant women upon admission to hospitals. Still an unknowing consent is not a valid consent, or a human act; and we the public can demand to know whether the medical profession means to use pregnant women in that way. The reason I would choose fully informed, truly voluntary consent to the application of any specific research procedure to the abortus is that it would require some discussion between the woman and her attending physician about the condemned fetus itself and its future, and not about the relief of her and her family's condition alone. If she does not change her mind about abortion—and I do not say that she should—I think it not likely that after full disclosure many understanding consents to abortus research would be forthcoming.

NOTES

INTRODUCTION

1. Barbara J. Culliton, "Grave-Robbing: The Charge against Four from Boston City Hospital," *Science, 186* (November 1, 1974), 420–23.

CHAPTER ONE

1. "The Use of Fetuses and Fetal Material for Research," Department of Health and Social Security, Scottish Home and Health Department, Welsh Office. London: Her Majesty's Stationery Office, 1972, hereafter referred to as the Peel Report.

2. G. R. Dunstan, *The Artifice of Ethics* (London: SCM Press, 1974), p. 53.

3. Ibid., p. 71, first italics added.

4. Bernard Häring, *Medical Ethics* (Notre Dame, Indiana: Fides Publications, 1972), pp. 75 ff.

5. These provisions are also summarized in "Research on Fetuses," *The Lancet* (June 3, 1972): 1222–23; and in the *British Medical Journal* (June 3, 1972): 550–51.

6. "Proposed Grant Code for Experiments on 'Viable Human Fetuses'," *Ob-Gyn News* (April 15, 1973).

7. Diana Copsey and Marion Gold, "NIH Ethics Policy Near on Fetal Research," *Ob-Gyn News* (April 15, 1973) (italics added).

8. "Issues in Draft Policy Debated in Council," *Ob-Gyn News* (April 15, 1973).

9. Harold M. Schmeck, Jr., "Research on Live Fetuses is Banned," The *New York Times,* April 18, 1973.

10. Michael T. Malloy, "A 'No' to Research on Aborted, Live Fetuses," The *National Observer,* April 12, 1973.

11. *Federal Register,* Vol. 38, No. 221 (Nov. 16, 1973), 31738–48. Below I refer to this document as the NIH guidelines or proposal; its revision, published in the *Federal Register,* vol. 39, No. 165 (Aug. 23, 1974), 30648–57, is referred to as the DHEW-NIH policy.

12. Amitai Etzioni, *Genetic Fix* (New York: Macmillan Publishing Co., 1973) is one such cry for help from a commission to tell us what to do.

13. "Issues in Draft Policy Debated in Council," *Ob-Gyn News* (April 15, 1973).

14. *Katie Relf, et al.* v. *Casper W. Weinberger, et al.,* Civil Action No. 73–1557, and *National Welfare Rights Organization* v. *Casper W. Weinberger, et al.,* Civil Action No. 74–243, U.S. District Court for the D.C.

15. *James R. Nielsen* v. *The Regents of the University of California, et al.,* No. 665–049, in the Superior Court of the State of California in and for the City and County of San Francisco.

16. Gary L. Reback, "Fetal Experimentation: Moral, Legal, and Medical Implications," *Stanford Law Review* (May 1974) 26: 1191–07, n. 135.

17. *Federal Register,* vol. 39, No. 165 (Aug. 23, 1974), pp. 30648–57, refered to below as the DHEW-NIH policy.

CHAPTER TWO

1. Geoffrey Chamberlain, "An Artificial Placenta," *American Journal of Obstetrics and Gynecology* (March 1, 1968), 100: 624.

2. See Paul Ramsey, *The Patient as Person* (New Haven: Yale University Press, 1970), p. 18.

3. "Live Abortus Research Raises Hackles of Some, Hopes of Others," *Medical World News* (October 5, 1973), pp. 32–36.

4. M. H. Pappworth, *Human Guinea Pigs* (Boston: Beacon Press, 1968).

5. LeRoy Walters, "Ethical Issues in Experimentation on the Human Fetus," *Journal of Religious Ethics,* (Spring 1974) 2: 33–54.

6. Anttis Vaheri, et al. "Isolation of Attenuated Rubella-Vaccine Virus from Human Products of Conception and Uterine Cervix." *New England Journal of Medicine* (May 18, 1972) 286: 1071–74.

7. Peter A. J. Adam et al., "Human Placental Barrier to [121]I-Glucagon Early in Gestation," *Journal of Clinical Endocrinology and Metabolism* (May 1972) 34: 772–82. See also Walters, pp. 35–36.

CHAPTER THREE

1. LeRoy Walters, "Ethical Issues in Experimentation on the Human Fetus," p. 48.

2. Ibid., p. 41.

CHAPTER FOUR

1. Jack Kevorkian, *Medical Research and the Death Penalty* (New York: Vantage Press, 1960); *Capital Punishment or Capital Gain?* (New York: Philosophical Library, 1962); "Capital Punishment or Capital Gain," *J. Crim. Law, Criminology and Police Science* (1959) 50: 50–51, Reprinted in Irving Ladimer and Roger W. Newman, eds., *Clinical Investigation in Medicine: Legal, Medical and Moral Aspects* (Boston University: Law-Medicine Research Institute, 1963), pp. 470–72; and in Jay Katz, et al., *Experimentation with Human Beings* (New York: Russell Sage Foundation, 1972), pp. 1027–28.

2. Kevorkian, "Capital Punishment or Capital Gain," pp. 50–51. Subsequent references are to this brief article, also in Ladimer, pp. 470–72, and Katz, pp. 1027–28.

3. Hans Jonas, "Philosophical Reflection on Human Experimentation," Ethical Aspects of Experimentation on Human Subjects, *Daedalus* (Spring 1969), 98: 241–43; reprinted in his *Philosophical Essays: From Ancient Creed to Technological Man* (Englewood Cliffs, N.J.: 1974), pp. 123–29.

4. Hans Jonas, *Philosophical Essays,* p. 126.

CHAPTER FIVE

1. "The Human Fetus as Useful Research Material," Case Studies in Bioethics, *Hastings Center Report* (April 1973) 3: 8–10. The discussants of this case were Dr. Robert S. Morison and Sumner B. Twiss, Jr. Subsequent references are to their debate about the ethics of this case.

2. "Issues in Draft Policy Debated in Council," *Ob-Gyn News* (April 15, 1973).

3. Willard Gaylin, M.D., and Marc Lappé, Ph.D., "Fetal Politics: The Debate on Experimenting with the Unborn," unpublished manuscript. Following quotations are from this article.

CHAPTER SEVEN

1. Walters, "Ethical Issues in Experimentation on the Human Fetus," p. 42.

2. Vaheri, et al., *NEJM* (1972) 286: 1071–74. See Chapter 2, above.

3. Agneta Philipson, L. D. Sabath, and David Charles. "Transplacental Passage of Erthromycin and Clindamycin," *New England Journal of Medicine* (June 7, 1973) 288: 1219–21.

4. International Code of Medical Ethics, adopted by the General Assembly of the World Medical Association, London, 1949.

5. *Jonas, Philosophical Essays*, p. 244.

CHAPTER EIGHT

1. Agneta Philipson *et al., NEJM* (1973) 288: 1219–21.

2. John A. Robertson, University of Wisconsin Law School, discusses this case in greater detail in "Medical Ethics in the Courtroom," *Hastings Center Report* (September 1974), 4:1–3. A single quotation from this important article is enough to indicate the legal and moral issues that may now be at trial and under judicial review. "Dr. Edelin can hardly argue in defense that his effort to shut off the fetus' blood supply before removal was justified as standard medical practice, for it

is the ethics of such practice which is being challenged. Resort to the legal system occurred because of the inability of the medical profession to engender sufficient consideration of fetal interests in late-term abortions." The abortus measured 21 centimeters from crown to rump and weighed 700 grams.

3. *Boston Globe,* April 23, 1974.

4. Barbara J. Culliton, "Grave-Robbing," *Science* (November 1, 1974), 420–23.

5. Gaylin and Lappé, "Fetal Politics."

6. Gary L. Reback, "Fetal Experimentation: Moral, Legal, and Medical Implications," *Stanford Law Review* (May 1974) 76: 1191–1207, n. 135.

CHAPTER NINE

1. Federal Register, vol. 39, No. 165, pp. 30648–57 (cited as the DHEW-NIH guidelines).

2. From a "Correction of Preamble to Proposed Policy," Protection of Human Subjects, issued by Casper W. Weinberger, *Federal Register,* vol. 39, No. 208 (October 21, 1974), p. 37993.

3. Ibid.

CHAPTER TEN

1. LeRoy Walters, p. 44.

2. Alexander Morgan Capron, "Legal Considerations Affecting Clinical Pharmacological Studies in Children," *Clinical Research* (February 1973), 141–50.